The Good Foot Book

Dedication

To my wife, Ruthie, and the three wonders of my life—my children Elyssa, Lauren, and Aaron.

Ordering

Trade bookstores in the U.S. and Canada please contact:

Publishers Group West
1700 Fourth Street, Berkeley CA 94710
Phone: (800) 788-3123   Fax: (510) 528-3444

Hunter House books are available at bulk discounts for textbook course adoptions; to qualifying community, health-care, and government organizations; and for special promotions and fund-raising. For details please contact:

Special Sales Department
Hunter House Inc., PO Box 2914, Alameda CA 94501-0914
Phone: (510) 865-5282   Fax: (510) 865-4295
E-mail: sales@hunterhouse.com

Individuals can order our books from most bookstores, by calling **(800) 266-5592,** or from our website at **www.hunterhouse.com**

The Good Foot Book

A Guide for Men, Women, Children, Athletes, Seniors — *Everyone*

Glenn Copeland, DPM, with Stan Solomon

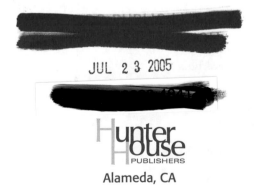

Hunter House
PUBLISHERS
Alameda, CA

> Hunter House Inc., Publishers
> PO Box 2914
> Alameda CA 94501-0914

Library of Congress Cataloging-in-Publication Data

Copeland, Glenn.
    The good foot book : a guide for men, women, children, athletes, seniors—everyone / Glenn Copeland with Stan Solomon.— 1st ed.
       p. cm.
    Includes index.
    ISBN 0-89793-448-2 (pbk.)
1. Foot—Care and hygiene. 2. Foot—Diseases—Popular Works. I. Solomon, Stan. II. Title.
RD563.C673 2004
617.5'85—dc22

                                                 2004016122

Project Credits

Illustrations: John Lightfoot
Cover Design: Peri Poloni, Knockout Books
Book Production: Rachel Reiss
Copy Editor: Kelley Blewster
Proofreader: John David Marion
Indexer: Nancy D. Peterson
Acquisitions Editor: Jeanne Brondino
Editor: Alexandra Mummery
Publishing Assistant: Antonia T. Lee
Publicist: Jillian Steinberger
Foreign Rights Coordinator: Elisabeth Wohofsky
Customer Service Manager: Christina Sverdrup
Order Fulfillment: Washul Lakdhon
Administrator: Theresa Nelson
Computer Support: Peter Eichelberger
Publisher: Kiran S. Rana

Manufactured in Canada by Transcontinental Printing

9 8 7 6 5 4 3 2 1   First Edition   05 06 07 08 09

Contents

Contents

Contents

Contents

List of Illustrations

Important Note

The material in this book is intended to provide a review of resources and information related to the prevention and treatment of certain foot and leg problems. Every effort has been made to provide accurate and dependable information. However, professionals in the field may have differing opinions and change is always taking place. Any of the treatments described herein should be undertaken only under the guidance of a licensed health-care practitioner. The author, editors, and publishers cannot be held responsible for any error, omission, professional disagreement, outdated material, or adverse outcomes that derive from the use of any of the treatments or information resources in this book, either in a program of self-care or under the care of a licensed practitioner.

Foreword

It is a genuine pleasure for me to write the Foreword to Glenn Copeland's new foot-care book. I welcome this opportunity as both a friend and a colleague, with admiration and much respect. As an author as well as a senior editor for numerous journals and textbooks, I have had the privilege to read wonderful scientific manuscripts, and to be able to recommend a popular health-care book in my field of interest and expertise is a real privilege. As a reader of this book, you are obviously seeking information, including answers to questions pertaining to basic but very common problems of the foot and ankle. These you will no doubt find here, written in an informative and comprehensive manner.

However, this is far more than "just another foot book," and I would like to take this opportunity to extend my warm congratulations to Glenn, the author. It is not easy to write a book. Indeed, it is an amazing accomplishment for any medical professional to write for both the scientific and lay public, as Glenn has done so successfully, at the same time juggling a busy clinical practice, as well as directing and managing a highly efficient and technologically advanced biomechanical program.

I have worked professionally with Glenn for the last four years and have been fortunate to develop a close professional and personal friendship with him. As an orthopedic surgeon with a specialized focus on the diagnosis and surgical correction of complex foot and ankle deformities, I always look to the basic "scientific roots" for a more complete knowledge of these complex deformities. Throughout *The Good Foot Book,* the how and why of the foot are wonderfully presented and discussed. The essence lies in an understanding of the biomechanics of the foot and ankle, in particular as it relates to the motion and propulsion of the human body—that is, how things work and, to some extent, how we stand, walk, and run—topics that Glenn has researched in depth for decades. He has spent the last twenty years developing new technologies to accurately measure and analyze both normal and abnormal functions of the foot, and is a recognized leader in this field.

Foreword

At the same time as our surgical skills and knowledge in our discipline have dramatically increased, so too have the diagnostic tools to measure foot function. We rely increasingly on technology for information, as well as an understanding of human function, and we owe much to leaders and innovators in the field, such as Glenn.

Glenn has introduced me to the more biomechanical aspects of gait and foot function, and I have been extremely fortunate to continue to learn from his former staff, who now work full-time in my institute as biomechanical and orthotic specialists. As an orthopedic surgeon, I want not only the best surgical care available for my patients, but also the best comprehensive foot care, including the biomechanical aspects of diagnosis now available to us. For a more comprehensive evaluation of patients and their problems, we now have access to highly sophisticated diagnostic equipment developed by Glenn. This has enabled us to treat patients more effectively, in particular maintaining a focus on understanding the biomechanical problems that underlie so many disorders of the foot and ankle. Whether a professional athlete or a homemaker, each patient has benefited from the state-of-the-art biomechanical diagnostic equipment that he has developed.

As Director of Mercy Medical Center's Institute for Foot and Ankle Reconstruction in Baltimore, Maryland, I strongly support any program of comprehensive care of the patient with foot and ankle problems, and throughout *The Good Foot Book* this philosophy is self-evident. I hope that, together with Glenn, we can continue to enhance patient care. With the technology that Glenn has introduced me to, we can continue to carry out comprehensive research on the causes of many foot and ankle problems, as well as their solutions. Sometimes the solution may be surgical, but with the recent technological advances, prevention of deformity—particularly in those who need it the most—is often possible. This is as important for the patient with diabetes who lacks feeling in the feet as it is for the professional athlete who is focused on performance.

On a more personal note, Glenn is a thoughtful, warm, and highly competitive individual who never loses perspective, and I am constantly touched by his caring and his intellect. His talents as a podiatrist, author, surgeon, and innovator are all in evidence in this marvelous book. I congratulate him on a most thorough, insightful, and articulate book for the public on the care and prevention of foot and ankle problems. I look forward to many years of enrichment and fulfillment in both my professional and personal relationships with him.

Mark Myerson, M.D.
Director, Institute for Foot and Ankle Reconstruction
Mercy Medical Center, Baltimore, Maryland

Acknowledgments

I have been most privileged to have had the opportunity to write four books. Those who have played major roles in this accomplishment have also been major supporters of many of my public and private endeavours. It is impossible to thank you all by name, but to my many friends and family, thank you for sharing my life.

I want to thank Meg Taylor and Clare McKeon at Key Porter Books; they have been huge supporters of this project and have been there for Stan and me with advice and guidance throughout the writing and revision processes. Thank you also to Gillian Watts for copyediting and Sue Sumeraj for proofreading.

Dr. Jeff Baker, Dr. Jack Barkin, Dr. Hamilton Hall, Dr. Ted Ross, Dr. Ron Taylor, and Dr. Robert Wolfe, renowned medical practitioners, educators, and wonderful care-givers, have been dear lifelong friends and colleagues who have helped and supported me through both the best and the trying times life throws at us. Dr. Robert Anderson, Dr. Hodges Davis, and Dr. Bruce Cohen, of the Miller Clinic in Charlotte, North Carolina, are all foot and ankle orthopedic surgeons who, early on, shared my vision of comprehensive foot care and helped develop the program outlined in this book. Dr. Johnny Lau, a foot and ankle orthopedic surgeon in Toronto, has been a great teacher in the newest surgical treatments for the foot and ankle.

Ernie Whitt and I met in 1977, when the Toronto Blue Jays were inaugurated. Ernie was an original Blue Jay who took me under his wing and introduced me to the world of professional baseball. Our families have grown up together and have shared many memorable experiences over the years. Ernie is a remarkable humanitarian who today spends most of his free time helping and supporting the Special Olympics. The friendship we share with Ernie and his bride of thirty years, Chris, has been a blessing.

I first met Shawn Green during spring training 1993, four weeks after the passing of my father. He carried himself then, as he does today, with great humility and grace. He adopted me as his friend and mentor almost immediately, and we have shared a very special and close relationship. Shawn and his wife, Lindsay, have become like my own children, and his wonderful parents, Ira and Judy, have included us as part of their family. I regret that my father, who taught me the love of baseball, didn't live long enough to meet Shawn.

Mark Myerson is a foot and ankle orthopedic surgeon who is considered one of the world's leading authorities in this area. We have spent many long hours together, discussing both professional and personal matters, and his guidance and input have really made this book possible. He continues to challenge me and teach me in all ways medical, and now even on the golf course, where he is down to a seven handicap. He is one person in medicine who would be difficult to emulate, as no single human I have ever met can approach his achievements. I am very proud and privileged that I can call him a friend, and I am humbled that he was so very generous in writing the Foreword for this book. He is what every young surgeon and professional aspires to but very few achieve.

I am not sure what my coauthor, Stan Solomon, did in his last life to deserve me, but it must have been horrendous. He has been my friend, student, teacher, confidant, babysitter, adviser, and supporter. He always understands why I am constantly forced to either cancel or show up for meetings an hour late. We all need a Stanley in our lives to bring calm when everything around us is out of control. None of my books would have been possible without his talents, patience, warmth, and understanding.

Introduction

Since my last book, *The Foot Doctor,* was published eight years ago, the diagnosis and treatment of foot problems have improved significantly, and with the appearance of ankle-replacement surgery we have entered a whole new era. In addition, an aging population and the explosion of medical information available over the Internet have altered the field considerably. After some discussion, my coauthor and I felt it was high time to write a new book.

First, I will mention the startling improvement in computerized gait analysis, which provides accurate assessment of existing and potential foot problems such as abnormal pronation. Abnormal pronation can result in a number of health problems—for example, bunions, hammer toes, plantar fasciitis, and even knee, hip, and back pain. This advance in assessment has led to a vast improvement in the design of orthotics (shoe inserts), which are used to prevent or treat such ailments. Moreover, these inserts can now be manufactured with new, lighter materials and can also be built directly into some shoes. This means that people who require orthotics are now able, for example, to wear sandals in the summer.

Treatment procedures have also improved markedly in the past four years. MRI (magnetic resonance imaging) examinations are now more readily available; these exams can reveal soft-tissue foot ailments that previously might have been missed or misdiagnosed unless more invasive procedures were used. New diagnostic ultrasound machines can easily pinpoint neuromas, tendonitis, and other soft-tissue problems that formerly could not be viewed by the available diagnostic means. New shockwave ultrasound machines can be used to treat ailments, such as plantar fasciitis and other forms of tendonitis, more effectively and efficiently than older treatment methods.

A revolutionary treatment that was unavailable until very recently is ankle-replacement surgery. I have had the privilege over the past few years to work with some of the world's most renowned foot and ankle surgeons. Dr. Mark Myerson of the Institute for Foot and Ankle Reconstruction at Mercy Medical Center,

Introduction

in Baltimore, Maryland, has generously contributed an explanation of how this most difficult surgery is performed. Although still in its infancy, ankle-replacement surgery will soon take its place beside hip and knee replacements.

A very active generation of baby boomers is reaching the wear-and-tear stage in life. In the coming years these people may well require professional foot care for many of the ailments I will be describing in this book. The streets, footpaths, and parks of our cities are flooded with runners—many of them baby boomers—early in the morning and late in the day, and from dawn to dusk on weekends. Most of them have been educated to wear proper running shoes, drink sufficient liquids, eat correctly, and stick to a disciplined training regimen. However, many of the older runners in particular are attempting to run distances for which their bodies—primarily their lower extremities—are not suited. Sooner or later they will wind up in a doctor's office, suffering from hip, knee, leg, ankle, or foot problems. As much as I applaud their efforts to stay fit, I would rather they listened to their bodies and sought the advice of a foot specialist at the first sign of trouble, rather than trying to tough it out. My office is filled with patients who followed exercise regimens, particularly those involving long-distance running, until they suffered serious problems.

There is also, unfortunately, another side to the baby-boomer coin: the couch potato who often develops systemic disorders related to inactivity and obesity that affect the feet. I am referring most specifically to those who develop circulatory or nerve disorders associated with cardiovascular disease and diabetes. Diabetics are especially prone to foot ulcers that, if left untreated (and occasionally even if treated), can lead to untreatable infections that result in amputation. Part of my job as a podiatrist is to ensure that my vulnerable patients remain intact, and I want to stress to my readers the importance of what I have to say in the chapters on systemic disorders and geriatrics.

The fourth major development since my last book is the explosion of medical information—both good and bad—on the Internet and in the media. Many doctors complain about patients asking for a specific drug or treatment they have read or heard about. I am all in favor of educated health-care consumers. However, some articles and advertisements can be unintentionally misleading or may fail to explain adequately to the nonprofessional the pros and cons of the treatments or prevention methods under discussion. Many articles in newspapers or on the Internet don't tell the whole story because of space constraints. Today drug companies are taking their advertising directly to the consumer via TV or Internet stories extolling the great virtues of their new drugs, but failing to cover in any detail the possible bad side effects. Far too many patients show up in the office demanding this or that drug, but only about 25 percent will accept a prescription after learning about the severe side effects. Patients must always weigh the risks and costs versus the benefits of taking any medication.

As far as articles on foot problems are concerned, I am quite skeptical of most that I read or hear. My skepticism is based on over thirty years of practice, and my belief that biomechanical faults in particular can be treated only with orthotics made specifically for that one person's feet. I pay more attention to articles on problems unrelated to biomechanical faults, especially if they offer me new information. For example, my coauthor showed me an Internet story regarding a "two-layer" dressing that supposedly helps diabetic foot ulcers heal. Since this dressing has been approved by the U.S. Food and Drug Administration to treat another condition, I believe it might be useful in the treatment of foot ulcers.

Drug advertising, which is more regulated in Canada than in the United States, is of particular concern to me. As I mentioned above, people who see an ad often fail to pay close enough attention to the possible serious side effects stated for the drug in question. Throughout this book I caution readers about the use of anti-inflammatory drugs because they can cause unrelated health problems. I am also careful when it comes to oral antifungal drugs. In the United States last year, a drug manufacturer was ordered to remove one of its television ads for an oral antifungal medication because it apparently failed to adequately explain to the public the potential serious side effects.

So my advice to the health-care consumer is *caveat emptor* (buyer beware). By all means, ask a medical professional about a certain drug or treatment, but don't insist on it if the expert has explained in depth why you won't benefit by using it. And listen closely to those TV ads when they rhyme off all the potential side effects of their drugs at the end of the commercial.

Occasionally a patient will tell me he or she has heard that fungal toenails can be treated by applying Listerine or Clorox, or that soaking tired feet in a heated wine-based solution will make them feel refreshed. There is no harm in trying these "old wives' remedies"—they often work quite well, although they may not be long-term solutions. And what I want for my patients is long-term relief, with no risk or downside. As we say in medicine, sometimes common sense is not very common.

Almost all biomechanical foot abnormalities can be prevented from becoming serious problems that require invasive treatment measures. I adhere to that old saying "an ounce of prevention is worth a pound of cure." I also emphasize that proper foot care will help prevent many of the lower-extremity maladies common today in both baby boomers and geriatrics, be they caused by biomechanical or by systemic disorders. I know that I must be doing something right, because many of my colleagues today are orthopedic specialists, particularly foot and ankle surgeons. When I first began practicing podiatry, very few orthopods were willing to accept me as a peer. I am happy to say that now many of us work together to provide our patients with the best possible care.

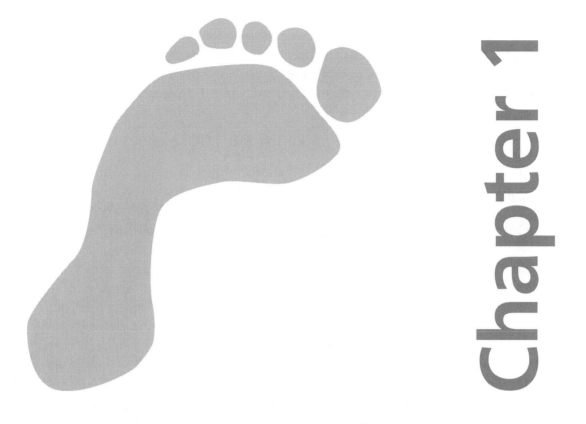

The Anatomy
of the Foot

Chapter 1: The Anatomy of the Foot

Readers familiar with my previous books may be tempted to skip these introductory chapters. Our understanding of the anatomy of the foot has not changed in the past few years, but it is worthwhile to review the information. When we get to the major themes of this book—prevention and treatment of specific foot and leg problems—then it will all make sense.

Many of my patients complain about the size and shape of their feet: They are either too big or too small, too wide or too narrow, too thick or too thin, or just plain fat and ugly. I have never understood why so many people hate their feet, or the feet of others. Even medical professionals voice such opinions. I once asked a doctor friend, "Just what is so disgusting about the human foot?"

"The size, shape, overall design, everything," he replied smugly. "It's total imperfection. But I guess that's why you chose podiatry. You must be making a fortune treating all those problems caused by bad feet."

I thought about his remarks for a few moments, then began to explain just how functional the foot really is. "First of all," I replied, "the foot has to act as a lever to propel the body." I then pointed out to him that the foot has to be flexible, and it must be able to turn in or out. It must also provide balance so that its owner doesn't keep falling over.

So my patients often dislike their "ugly" feet, and my medical colleagues tend to view the foot with disdain. All the more reason for me to put the foot on a pedestal and to convince people to put aesthetics aside and learn how the foot functions and why it is shaped the way it is.

What's a-Foot?

A foot is, or ought to be, the most dependable form of transportation you have, and it can often be an excellent barometer of your general physical condition. Imagine that your body is a finely tuned automobile, and that your feet are the wheels. (In fact, athletes often refer to their lower extremities as "wheels.") If your wheels are out of alignment, your total performance suffers. Conversely, as you will see in later chapters, trouble elsewhere in your body can manifest itself in your feet.

We will return to the analogy of your body as a machine later, but first I want to illustrate, in words and with diagrams, the anatomy of the foot—the bones and joints, the muscles and tendons, the ligaments, cartilage, blood vessels, and nerves. Once I have dealt with the parts of the foot, I will proceed to illustrate in the next chapter how they all work together to enable you to walk, run, jump, dance, play, or do whatever else you wish while on your feet.

A Quick Course in Anatomy

A human foot, ugly or beautiful, is not always 12 inches long. Foot size in a normal, healthy adult can range from 4½ inches long by 3 inches wide (11 x 8 cm) to 24

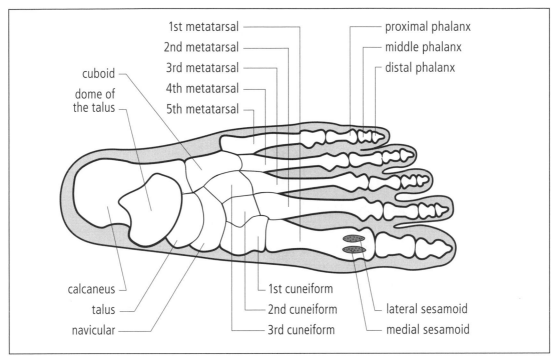

Figure 1.1. Bones of the foot

inches long by 9 inches wide (61 x 23 cm). In most cases feet are made to order for your particular body shape and size. Exceptionally tall women often complain to me about their difficulty in finding attractive shoes to fit what they consider to be huge, unattractive feet. However, these women would look very silly with size 5 or 6 feet. Moreover, they would be unable to balance themselves properly, and would probably blow over in high winds. I advise these women to complain to shoe designers and manufacturers for satisfaction, rather than complaining about their fate.

Medical geniuses long ago divided the foot into three distinct parts: the *forefoot,* from the tips of the toes to the base of the metatarsals (the five bones that connect the midfoot and rearfoot bones to the toe bones); the *midfoot,* including the cuneiform, cuboid, and navicular bones; and the *rearfoot,* including the talus (ankle) and calcaneus (heel) bones (see Figure 1.1). Many people refer to the "ball" of the foot and the "arch" without knowing exactly where they are located. The ball is considered to be in the forefoot—on the bottom of the foot, under the metatarsal heads. The arch is generally considered to be in the midfoot area.

It is an interesting fact, at least to me, that over 95 percent of all foot surgery is done on the forefoot. However, these days many foot problems occur in the heel and ankle areas. I will explain why in various chapters throughout the book, but if you guess that it has to do with baby boomers who have been subjecting their bodies to stressful athletic endeavors for years, you will have hit the nail on the head.

Bones

You may be surprised to learn that a quarter of all the bones in the human body are in the feet. The normal foot has twenty-six bones of varying sizes and shapes (see Figure 1.1), plus two sesamoids, which lie underneath the first metatarsal. However, it is not uncommon for a person to have small extra bones called *accessory ossicles*. These extra bones are thought to be hereditary, and seldom cause any trouble. For anyone to have too few bones in the foot would be a medical rarity.

Bones and biomechanics go together, as you will learn in the following chapter. Getting back to our analogy of the body as a machine, you know that when one cog in a wheel is misshapen, the wheel, and hence the machinery, will malfunction. The same holds true for the foot when one of its bones is defective. An abnormal bone can lead to a biomechanical fault.

But before we get to biomechanical details, we have to examine other parts of the foot: the joints; all the soft tissues that hold the bones and joints in place and facilitate their movement, such as muscles, tendons, cartilage, and ligaments; the supply system that lubricates and nourishes the bones and soft tissues; and the electrical, or nerve, system that transmits signals to and from the brain, telling the feet when and where to go.

Joints

Two or more bones that come together *articulate* to form a joint. We hear a great deal about joints when we discuss arthritis and cartilage problems, and they can be a terrible pain at times. But without joints we would be quite inflexible, because most of them move, at least slightly, to allow our bodies to assume different postures and motions.

The joint in the foot that you probably think about most is the ankle joint, which connects the lower part of the leg to the back of the foot. It is a hinge-type joint in that its motion resembles that of a door opening. When you damage an ankle joint, walking or running becomes a nightmare because of the pain that occurs when weight is placed on the foot. Your gait can become exaggerated as you attempt to compensate by forcing most of the weight onto the other foot during the walking cycle. As a result, the biomechanics of both feet can be adversely affected.

A more crucial joint affecting the biomechanics of the foot during walking or running is the *subtalar* joint. It comprises three different articulations between the top surface of the heel bone and the bottom surface of the ankle bone. As you will see in the following chapter, when a person pronates (rolls from the outside of the heel inward) abnormally, the subtalar joint does not move as it should. If this occurs, a chain reaction develops and problems can occur throughout the foot.

The *midtarsal* joint, in the arch area of the foot, works together with the subtalar joint to help the foot compensate for a biomechanical fault, particularly a temporary one. This could occur when walking or running on uneven terrain or when upper-body motion changes—for example, when an athlete or a dancer assumes an unusual position. When the subtalar and midtarsal joints cannot compensate adequately for a more long-lasting biomechanical fault, the result could be a foot disorder. The subtalar joint used to be blamed for such disorders,

but since computer and camera techniques that measure foot motion have become so much better in the past four years, we now know that the midtarsal joint is the leading culprit in forefoot compensation.

People are unlikely to suffer to any great extent from subtalar or midtarsal joint pain. However, one other type of joint in the foot can cause excruciating pain at times: the *metatarso-phalangeal* joint. Five of these joints are formed by articulation of the heads of the metatarsal bones (in the ball area of the foot) and the ends of the proximal phalanges (the large bones in the toes). These joints can be seen in Figure 1.2.

Figure 1.2. Joints of the foot and ankle

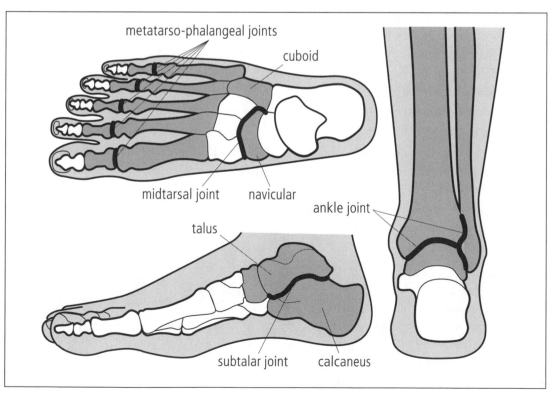

For reasons that I will describe in subsequent chapters, the big-toe joint—where the proximal phalanx (the big bone of the first, or great, toe) and the metatarsal head come together—often bears the brunt of unequal weight distribution that a biomechanical fault inflicts on the foot. As a result, this joint is subjected to a lot of added wear and tear that makes it susceptible to osteoarthritis and similar conditions. Gout may also affect the big-toe joint, but this is not caused by a biomechanical problem. As you will discover in Chapter 10, gout is a disease that can be controlled by proper medication and diet.

Although there are many other joints in the foot, our major concern in this book is the four joints mentioned above, because they are the ones that most affect, and are affected by, biomechanical foot faults. However, it is not uncommon to have problems with the *interphalangeal* joints, which lie between the phalanges, or toe bones, in the various toes (two bones comprise the big toe, and all the other toes have three bones). When I discuss forefoot pain in Chapter 4, I will deal with conditions that can affect these phalangeal joints.

Muscles

There are nineteen individual muscles in the foot and lower leg that interconnect to help move the foot. Simply put, when muscles are overstressed or otherwise abnormal, they can affect the biomechanics of the foot because they can pull tendons and bones out of place and irritate joints. Conversely, a bone defect can cause muscle injury. I will discuss damage to particular muscles of the foot in great detail in subsequent chapters. I will also describe—particularly in Chapters 11 and 12, which deal with athletic activities—how muscles in the leg can affect or be affected by the biomechanics of the feet during various types of physical activities.

The Connectors

Tendons attach muscles to bones. Actually they are extensions of muscles. They are tough whitish cords that are somewhat elastic and flexible. When a muscle has been stretched to its maximum potential, the force of the stretch is transferred to the tendon. The tendon itself may then become overstretched, and the result is *tendonitis*, or inflammation of the tendon.

Ligaments are thick, inelastic, but slightly flexible structures that support and surround the joints, holding bone to bone. When an ankle is twisted or a big toe is stubbed, the cause of the discomfort and swelling is usually a ligament that has been overstretched or slightly torn.

Cartilage

Cartilage is dense connective tissue that serves as a lining on the ends of bones where they meet to form joints. If you look at the end of a chicken drumstick, you will notice white gristle lining the bone. That white gristle is cartilage.

Cartilage provides smooth surfaces between bones. Without cartilage, your body would literally grind to a halt. Your joints would make a terrible racket when you moved as bone ground against bone. You would also be in severe pain from inflammation in the joints caused by the bones grinding together.

In Circulation

Two main arteries supply the feet with the necessary blood: the *dorsalis pedis* artery and the *posterior tibial* artery. These major arteries spread oxygenated blood via smaller *arterioles* to the many tissues of the feet. If the arterial system fails to supply the life-supporting oxygen contained in the red blood cells, serious problems could result.

Because the major foot arteries are the farthest from the heart of any in the human body, many circulatory problems will first manifest themselves in the feet. Two examples are *arteriosclerosis* (hardening of the arteries) and *atherosclerosis* (a buildup of plaque inside the arteries, leading to their subsequent blockage).

We all know that veins are the vessels that return used blood to the heart and lungs for regeneration—that is, to obtain a new supply of nutrients and oxygen— after the blood's supply of oxygen has been used to nourish the tissues of the body. Two sets of veins return blood from the lower extremities to the heart and lungs. The superficial veins, which run close to the surface of the skin and move spent (deoxygenated) blood from the feet to the heart and lungs, are the *great saphenous*—the longest vein in the body, running up the big-toe side of the foot and along the inside of the leg—and the *small saphenous,* which runs along the outside part of the foot and up the back of the leg. The deep veins, farther below the surface of the skin, are the *anterior tibial* and the *posterior tibial.* The position of the saphenous veins can be seen in Figure 1.3. Incidentally, it is the great saphenous vein that heart surgeons sometimes use in bypass surgery.

Figure 1.3. Veins of the leg

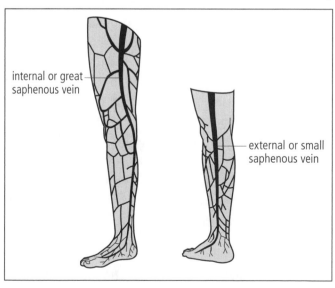

internal or great saphenous vein

external or small saphenous vein

Then there are tiny auxiliary veins *(venuoles),* which are the opposite of the arterioles that deliver fresh blood to various more remote areas of the body. The venuoles pick up used blood from the nether reaches of the feet and deliver it to the larger veins for the journey up to the heart and lungs. *Capillaries* are the crossover links between the arterioles and the venuoles.

People with circulatory problems in their lower extremities often complain of swollen ankles, a condition that worsens after a long day on one's feet or after a lengthy airplane flight. The majority of such problems, including varicose veins, are related to poor venous (vein) function in the feet. Treatments do exist for such conditions, and they will be described in detail in Chapter 10.

Podiatrists, and other medical professionals who are on their toes, will examine the feet of their patients for any changes in skin color, texture, and temperature. Such changes can be tip-offs to certain circulatory problems that will be described in Chapter 10. But I will tell you now that it is unwise to make any diagnoses yourself. If one of your toes looks and feels funny, don't assume that this indicates serious cardiovascular disease and go into a panic. See your doctor at once for a more reliable opinion.

On Your Nerves

Nerves supply feeling and muscle control to particular parts of the body, the foot being one of them. It has four major nerves to provide you with many weird and wonderful sensations. These four nerves are the *posterior tibial,* the *superficial peroneal,* the *deep peroneal,* and the *sural.*

Nerve problems in the foot are commonly related to compression syndromes—that is, a nerve is being pinched or squeezed. For example, an improperly fitting shoe can put so much pressure on a nerve that the area around the nerve swells. This causes *nerve entrapment,* which in turn can lead to pain and numbness, and occasionally to a strange, seemingly unrelated discomfort that I call "enigmatic pain." Nerve disorders in other parts of the body—for example, sciatica—can also have manifestations in the feet. These and other nerve diseases that affect the lower extremities will be discussed in various chapters throughout the book.

Functions of the Foot

Now that we know the roles of the major components of the foot, before we proceed to the chapter on biomechanics, we ought to briefly examine the functions of the foot. It is important to know what the foot does in order to be able to understand why its proper range of motions is so vital in keeping you on an even keel when you are walking or running.

First, the mobile foot helps you adapt to certain ground surfaces. If you have trouble adapting to walking or running on hard, soft, wet, or dry surfaces, you may fall flat on your face. The foot functions much as the tires of a car do to assure a smooth, safe ride on various terrains.

Second, the foot is a rigid lever that propels the body forward—and in other directions. Without this function you would have great difficulty maneuvering your body in any direction.

Third, the foot is a shock absorber that absorbs most of the stress to which your body is subjected while you are on your feet. If the foot did not perform this function, other shock-absorbing areas of the body,

such as the knees and the spinal column, would be under extreme stress that would cause early wear and tear on their joints.

The fact that the human foot accomplishes these three feats is actually quite amazing. As one of my professors said to me years ago, "It's not the problems of the foot that intrigue me as much as what the foot is capable of withstanding during the course of a normal lifetime." So, with all due respect to my medical colleagues and most of my patients, I intend to prove to you that the foot is not a monstrosity after all.

Chapter 2

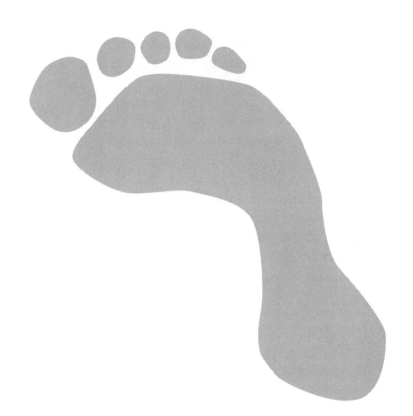

The Biomechanics of the Foot and Lower Leg

The study of human biomechanics is still relatively new, but it has made rapid strides since it was kick-started by the jogging craze in the late 1970s. It was runners with "overuse" syndromes—problems caused by constant normal and/or abnormal forces on the feet over long periods of time—that convinced previously skeptical medical practitioners that the foot is indeed the culprit in many lower-limb and back ailments. Over the years that I have been podiatric consultant at Mount Sinai Hospital's Sports Medicine Clinic in Toronto, my colleagues and I have concluded, in particular, that many complaints from the knee down are directly related to poor mechanical function of the lower leg and foot.

To understand how many foot and lower-leg problems begin, you must have a grasp of the mechanics of a person's gait—in simple terms, the way you walk, run, or play. Some of you may become stressed when you hear the word *mechanics* because you have trouble even fitting two Lego pieces together. But rest assured, understanding the biomechanics of the foot in motion is not that difficult.

To begin with, foot problems have occurred since our ancestors started walking on two legs. Most mammals have at least four appendages to walk on, and, biomechanically, walking on four legs is much easier on the lower limbs and spinal column than walking on two. Compared to our four-legged cousins, humans have more difficulty walking or running on dif-

ferent terrains and surfaces, and therefore must have extremely adaptive lower extremities—particularly the foot—in order to remain upright and move efficiently and effectively. When humans have trouble with their feet while walking or running, the problems usually stem from poor biomechanics.

I have simplified the details because an exhaustive examination of the mechanics of walking or running requires extensive knowledge in various related fields—for example, medicine, physics, kinesiology, and ergonomics. Also, a complete treatment of the subject would take a few hundred pages. What I have tried to do is help you understand how your foot moves, and how certain disorders of the foot and lower limbs can be caused either directly or indirectly by biomechanical faults. You will need this information to be able to understand much of the material in the following chapters.

What Is Biomechanics?

Biomechanics refers to the study of human motion—for our purposes specifically, the motions of the foot and leg in stride. The graceful motions of a ballet dancer or a runner in full, fluid stride provide suitable examples of essentially flawless biomechanics in action. Perhaps the prime example of perfect biomechanics would be a champion racehorse in full flight down the home stretch, but this is a book about humans, not about Seabiscuit.

Chapter 2: The Biomechanics of the Foot and Lower Leg

It is only within the past four decades that podiatrists have joined the forefront of researchers seeking to understand abnormal walking and running motions. They did this in order to treat foot disorders they deemed to be caused by biomechanical faults. Indeed, successful treatments have resulted from their newfound ability to investigate the forces, both normal and abnormal, that press on the foot when it is bearing weight. A by-product of this progress is our ability today to deal successfully with foot problems that have been shown to affect other parts of the body, from the lower back to the ankle. Remember that song about the foot bone being connected to the leg bone, and on up the body? Well, it is definitely true that problems with foot bones can adversely affect backbones, and all the other bones in between.

Abnormal Biomechanics

The overwhelming majority of lower-limb problems that are not related to injury, and a fair number of lower-back, knee, and hip complaints, are caused by abnormal biomechanics of the foot and/or leg. A large percentage of these problems can be successfully treated with special shoe inserts: orthotics. As you will learn below, we are now able, with the help of computers, to provide accurate diagnosis and orthotic treatment of most biomechanical abnormalities.

As we discuss abnormal biomechanics, it will help to recall the main functions of the foot so that we understand how these abnormalities can adversely affect your physical well-being.

- First, a normal foot functions much as a tire does on a car to assure a smooth, safe ride on various terrains. If the tire (or the foot) wears on one side or develops irregularities, the ride can become uneven, and eventually unpleasant; the entire car (or body) can become out of alignment. Starting from the moment of heel contact, the foot acts as a mobile adapter to adjust to the surface that it is striking.

- Second, the foot is a rigid lever that propels the body forward or helps it change direction. An abnormal foot can cause great difficulty in maneuvering the body in any direction, because the normal foot has a much greater range of motion than the hip or knee. It is the basic compensatory part of the lower limb.

- Third, when a person is in stride, the foot is a shock absorber. If the foot fails to perform this function adequately, other parts of the body, such as the knees, hips, or lower back, have to take up the slack. This added stress eventually results in early wear and tear to the joints of these body parts—for example, painful osteoarthritis.

When we speak of the walking or gait cycle, we are referring to a person's range of motions when moving forward. A normal complete cycle is divided into two separate phases: swing and stance. *Swing* is when the foot is off the ground. However, the *stance* phase—when the foot is in contact with the ground—is the part of the cycle that we are most concerned about. The stance phase accounts for 65 percent of the cycle. In other words, each foot is on the ground 65 percent of the time during the cycle, not 50 percent—we would walk rather strangely if only one foot were on the ground with each step we took.

The stance phase of the gait cycle is divided into three segments: heel-strike, mid-stance, and propulsion (see Figure 2.1). As you would expect, foot and foot-related problems arise when something goes wrong during the stance phase—most often during mid-stance, when the body weight is being distributed across the mid-foot. When a biomechanical fault occurs, an abnormal amount of weight is brought

to bear on a specific part of the foot. When we discuss specific problems below, you will see how such abnormalities adversely affect the foot and other parts of the body, and how we can determine which abnormality causes discomfort at a certain point.

During the first segment (heel-strike) of the stance phase of the gait cycle, the foot naturally pronates (rolls from the outside of the heel inward). This is why it is normal for the heel of the shoe to wear down on the outside. In mid-stance the foot is in a neutral position, and then it begins to supinate (roll toward the outside of the foot) during the latter part of the stance phase, from the beginning of propulsion to when the foot lifts off the ground.

A full 98 percent of all biomechanical foot problems are caused by abnormal

Figure 2.1. The gait cycle

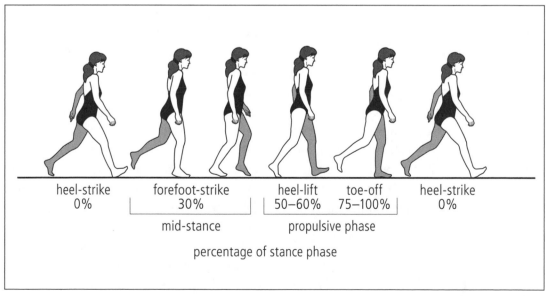

| heel-strike 0% | forefoot-strike 30% | | heel-lift 50–60% | toe-off 75–100% | heel-strike 0% |

mid-stance   propulsive phase

percentage of stance phase

pronation; the other 2 percent are caused by the opposite motion, supination. Since many cases of abnormal supination are caused by neuromuscular disorders that require treatment by a specialist, in this chapter, and throughout the book, we shall be concentrating primarily on abnormal pronation.

Basically, 25 percent of the stance phase is the first segment (heel-strike), the second segment (mid-stance) is 50 percent, and the third segment (propulsion) is 25 percent. This may explain why more abnormal pronation takes place during the second segment. Abnormal pronation occurs when a foot either pronates when it should be in a neutral position or supinating, or overpronates during the normal pronation period of the gait cycle.

Let us follow the gait cycle through its stance phase. From heel-strike almost to the beginning of the second segment (mid-stance), the subtalar joint in a normal foot pronates up to 4 degrees. The joint then moves to a neutral position (zero degrees) in the mid-stance. At the beginning of the propulsion segment, it moves to about 4 degrees of supination, which it maintains until the end of the stance phase. During the swing phase the subtalar joint is in a neutral position, but it begins to pronate again at heel-strike. Problems occur when the subtalar joint pronates abnormally. We shall discuss below why this abnormality can occur.

The midtarsal joint also plays a pivotal role in the stance phase, specifically during mid-stance, when it receives the weight of the person in stride. If the subtalar joint is abnormally pronating, the midtarsal joint attempts to correct the situation. However, when the heel-strike is abnormal, that abnormal motion can flow through the midfoot to the forefoot and, depending on the degree of the abnormality, the midtarsal joint may be unable to compensate fully.

Imagine a line that begins at the back of the heel, moves through the center of the midfoot, and ends approximately between the big and second toe. This line represents normal weight distribution on the foot during the stance phase of the gait cycle. Any significant deviation from that line almost always indicates abnormal pronation. Various abnormal pronation patterns cause different parts of the feet to be overstressed by being forced to accept an abnormal amount of weight. The effects of abnormal pronation may be felt in several places in the body.

Before the computerized measurement system discussed below was developed, we were unable to determine exactly where and to what degree an abnormality was actually occurring. Such an understanding is critical in effectively treating problems related to biomechanics, because static measurements of the foot fail to pinpoint the precise areas where dysfunction occurs. As you will soon see, we now understand, for example, how a bunion forms (tight shoes exacerbate the condition rather than cause it), which means that it

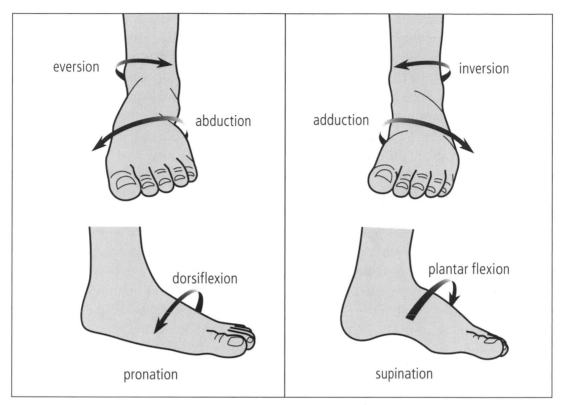

Figure 2.2. Pronation and supination

can be either prevented or treated before surgery becomes necessary.

Pronation and Supination

We shall return shortly to the gait cycle and abnormal biomechanics of the foot. But first it is time to define the terms *pronation* and *supination* more fully, because you will be reading a lot about them in this book. Eventually I will be talking more specifically about how abnormal pronation and supination can cause foot disorders, but at this point I want you to understand that normal feet do pronate and supinate a certain amount during the stance phase of the

gait cycle. So when you hear that someone pronates, it is an abnormal pronation syndrome that is being referred to.

The foot naturally pronates during the first part (contact) of the stance phase of the gait cycle. Pronation involves three distinct motions of the foot during this phase (see Figure 2.2). These motions all occur simultaneously and are called *eversion, abduction* (not to be confused with kidnapping), and *dorsiflexion*. These terms may seem obscure to most people, but do not feel discouraged by your lack of knowledge. The average medical student may graduate from medical school and set up practice without ever truly understanding their meanings—or the full meanings of *pronation* and *supination,* for that matter.

Supination is the exact opposite of pronation. The opposing biomechanical movements of the foot are *inversion, adduction,* and *plantar flexion.* Supination occurs normally during the latter part of the stance phase, from the beginning of the propulsion stage to when the foot lifts off the ground.

As mentioned earlier, abnormal pronation—the major cause of foot problems— occurs when a foot pronates when it should be supinating, or overpronates during a normal pronation period of the gait cycle. A foot supinates abnormally when it ought to be pronating, or when it exceeds a normal amount of supination. As we follow the foot through the gait cycle, keep in mind that some pronation and supination are necessary at certain times to enable the foot to propel forward properly, but only up to about 4 degrees each. Another important aspect to remember is that when the foot is neither pronating nor supinating, it is in the neutral position. If the foot is pronating or supinating during the stance phase of the gait cycle when it ought to be in the neutral position, a biomechanical problem may exist.

The subtalar joint works with the midtarsal joint to compensate for temporary pronation or supination problems caused by external factors such as uneven terrain, or by a change in upper-body motion—for example, when an athlete kicks a ball or a ballet dancer does a pirouette. When these joints are unable to compensate for a continuous and/or acute biomechanical problem, a foot disorder can develop.

The main stress on the midtarsal joint occurs when the foot is in the mid-stance stage of the stance phase. It becomes more difficult for the midtarsal joint to compensate for a biomechanical problem when the first stage of the stance phase is abnormal and cannot be corrected by the subtalar joint. So, if you land abnormally on your foot at heel-strike, the effects of the fault may flow all the way through to the forefoot, where it may manifest itself as a metatarsal-head or toe-joint disorder. The result could be anything from a bunion to a callus or a corn, depending on just where the abnormal amount of weight is being brought to bear.

Abnormal Pronation

Abnormal compensatory pronation is the most common cause of foot disorders. Although there are many reasons why the foot might pronate abnormally, in my patients I see five causes (mentioned below) far more than any others. Keep in mind that when a foot has a biomechanical fault, an excessive amount of weight may be focused on a particular part of the foot. It is this overstressing of that part of the foot that causes problems, as nature reacts to protect the stressed area, often by forming a layer of protective skin that itself can become irritated, or at other times by deviating a bone or a soft-tissue mass. Let me also emphasize that the biomechanical faults that cause foot disorders are usually congenital; that is, the person is born with an abnormality or with a propensity to develop one.

The five most common causes of abnormal pronation are forefoot varus, forefoot valgus, a rearfoot varus deformity (see Figure 2.3), subtalar varus, and lack of motion in the ankle joint. Let me assure you that these conditions are hardly life-threatening (one of the joys of being a podiatrist is that I never get emergency calls in the middle of the night) and do not require painful, lengthy treatments to ameliorate. They are simply bony abnormalities that commonly create abnormal pronation.

Problems in the lower leg can also cause the foot to pronate abnormally, such as tibial varum (bow legs), internal tibial or femoral torsion, a short Achilles tendon or calf muscle, short hamstring or iliopsoas

Figure 2.3. Abnormal pronation

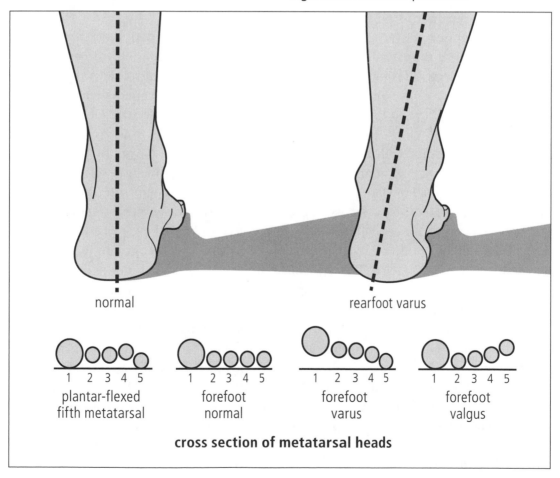

normal

rearfoot varus

1 2 3 4 5	1 2 3 4 5	1 2 3 4 5	1 2 3 4 5
plantar-flexed fifth metatarsal	forefoot normal	forefoot varus	forefoot valgus

cross section of metatarsal heads

muscles, or a discrepancy in lower limb length. These problems may go unnoticed until you decide to take up an athletic endeavor. As you will learn in Chapters 11 and 12, certain physical activities will bring to the fore biomechanical faults in the leg and foot that otherwise might not cause any trouble.

As I have mentioned, the primary reason why it is so important to avoid abnormal pronation or supination is that a biomechanical fault can cause an abnormal amount of force to be focused on one part of the foot. Continuous excessive weight brought to bear on one area of the foot will eventually cause a problem at that site, as you will learn in the following chapters.

Abnormal Supination

Abnormal supination will receive short shrift in this book, as it accounts for only a small percentage of all the foot problems I have seen in my years as a podiatrist, and I am sure that my practice is no different from those of my podiatrist colleagues throughout North America. The typical supinating foot is one with a very high arch and a rigid structure (see Figure 2.2), and the problem causing the supination syndrome may have a neuromuscular component.

Although I can diagnose a biomechanical fault such as a patient's overpronation with my naked eye, I am not a computer or some other high-tech diagnostic tool. Therefore I cannot measure precisely the exact amount of pronation in a foot at a given point in the gait cycle. However, computerized diagnostic equipment available today has revolutionized examination of the gait cycle so that adjustments, in the form of an orthotic insert fitted into the shoe, can be made to correct a fault. I will discuss this new equipment and orthotics shortly.

Examining for a Biomechanical Foot Fault

Once foot specialists have learned the tricks of the trade, their trained eyes can catch many foot faults. I can judge the relationships between patients' feet and legs by watching them walk barefoot on a flat surface, and can determine visually whether or not they are abnormally pronating or supinating. So, while no two feet are alike, some are far enough from the norm that their idiosyncrasies can be spotted by the experienced naked eye.

The two most common features of an abnormally shaped foot are the high arch (pes cavus) and the low arch (pes planus). The high-arched foot is often, but not always, somewhat rigid, and it is a poorer shock absorber than the normal arch. Because of its shape, the metatarsal heads of the foot (the ends of the metatarsal bones that articulate with the toe bones) are exposed to added pressure when the forefoot is bearing weight. Numerous forefoot disorders can result, although many people with high-arched feet are fine unless they take up an activity or wear shoes that put even more stress on the forefoot during the walking cycle.

The Myth of Flat Feet and Fallen Arches

I always avoid corny jokes about flat feet and fallen arches. So-called flat feet have been used as an excuse by artful draft dodgers to avoid military service in the various countries where it is compulsory. There are also numerous anecdotes and jokes about "flatfoots"—policemen who have walked the beat for too long—and dim-witted or slow-moving individuals who have been "caught flat-footed." So, despite attempts by the medical profession to correct faulty information—or perhaps with its help on occasion—the flat foot and the fallen arch have become widely accepted concepts, much like the slipped disc. But feet are hardly ever completely flat, and arches do not fall. In fact, the world-renowned Mayo Clinic newsletter recently suggested that all those exemptions from military service for flat feet were misguided; the high-arched rigid foot is much more the culprit in foot and lower leg problems.

True flat feet are congenital, and they are rarely seen. The low-arched foot is not necessarily abnormal, and it is definitely *not* flat. However, the shape of the foot makes it tend to overpronate during the gait cycle,

and as a result it appears flat when weight is brought to bear on it (see Figure 2.2).

How a Biomechanical Fault Can Cause a Foot Disorder

Now you understand the fundamental biomechanics of the motions of the foot as it goes through the walking cycle. Motion flows down the leg, through the ankle and the subtalar joint, through the midtarsal joint, and all the way down to and across the metatarsal heads to the big toe. Let me illustrate now how a biomechanical fault can occur, perhaps because of a congenital foot abnormality, and how it can affect everything from the forefoot all the way up to the lower back.

In the abnormal foot—the toes of which are shown in cross-section in Figure 6.1 on page 65—the second metatarsal bone (the second-largest bone in the forefoot) is closer to the ground than the other four metatarsal bones. This is true for both a high-arched and a low-arched foot. As a result, more pressure is being applied to the second metatarsal during the latter part of the stance phase of the gait cycle than to the other metatarsal bones. Because that bone bears excessive weight, it will eventually become inflamed. This sets off a chain reaction. A callus will form on the skin under the bone, causing it to become even more inflamed and bruised, both from the pounding it is receiving and from the stress of the callus.

Eventually the pain in the area will become severe enough that the victim will try to compensate by shifting weight to the baby-toe side of the foot, thereby creating an abnormal supination syndrome. This imbalanced, abnormal gait will affect the biomechanics of the entire foot and leg and can create discomfort on the outside of the knee and even in the hip. This is because all the muscles and tendons in those areas are being overextended and the knee and hip joints are therefore also becoming inflamed.

Once the original problem—the abnormally positioned second metatarsal bone—is treated, the biomechanics of the lower extremities should normalize. If the conditions have not been allowed to go on for too long, all the symptoms will disappear.

The above example illustrates how a foot problem can adversely affect other parts of the body. Of course, this syndrome can also operate in reverse. An abnormal calf muscle can place added strain on the Achilles tendon, and subsequently on the ankle joint. This could create an abnormal pronation problem in the subtalar joint—a biomechanical fault that did not begin in the foot. As a result, added pressure may be put on one part of the foot when it is bearing weight, and an inflammation could develop.

Arthritis

Abnormal pronation and supination can often lead to osteoarthritis. There is much discussion in medical circles today as to whether osteoarthritis is a wear-and-tear disorder, a systemic disease, or both. Why, for example, do some athletes develop osteoarthritis in severely stressed joints, while others do not? I leave that argument to the researchers. However, I do know that a simple wear-and-tear process in any joint of the body can precipitate an inflammation because of breakdown of the cartilage tissue that normally keeps bone from rubbing against bone. Cartilage tissue can be unduly stressed and broken down by abnormal forces in the joint, forces that often result from a biomechanical fault in the lower limbs.

If an athlete or a dancer regularly places excessive stress on the lower limbs while exercising or performing, the joints in the lower extremities of the body will be subjected to more wear and tear than the joints of people who do not partake in strenuous activity. It is not disease that is damaging or destroying the stressed joints, but normal external, but excessive, biomechanical forces. Would you expect even the best tires to last forever on a racing car? Even on a normal car, an excellent set of tires will have to be replaced after fifty thousand to seventy-five thousand miles. The tires are neither diseased nor faulty, just worn down. The same applies to the joints in our bodies. However, we often help speed up the degeneration process by allowing a biomechanical fault or excessive stress to continue until the joint has been sufficiently inflamed to cause discomfort and, eventually, dysfunction. When you allow a biomechanical fault to continue untreated, you are helping along the wear-and-tear process in the joints of your feet, legs, hips, and lower back, because you are constantly placing undue stress on those joints in order to walk or run.

About 90 percent of all common foot pain, including osteoarthritis, is caused by abnormal biomechanical forces. And, just as faulty wheel alignment in a car can result in tire wear and tear, the abnormal forces caused by misalignment in your lower limbs can cause early wear and tear of the joints in your feet. As we have already discussed, foot problems can create havoc in the entire bottom half of your body. However, with proper mechanical adjustments—for example, the wearing of orthotics—further wear and tear can be prevented and pain can be drastically reduced, or even eliminated altogether in many cases.

There are other forms of arthritis—rheumatoid, gouty, and psoriatic, to name the most common of them—that are called *systemic arthritic diseases*. They are caused by internal disorders that can, unlike osteoarthritis, be classified as diseases. Less than half of one percent of my "arthritic" patients suffer from the systemic disease varieties. I will discuss the more common of these diseases in Chapter 10.

Orthotics

The last thing I want to mention in this chapter is the orthotic device that fits into a shoe. It is designed to properly redistribute the weight on the foot and to correct any abnormal foot motions.

Custom-made leather inserts have been found in footwear made as far back as the fifteenth century. In those days, all boots and shoes were made by hand, and the shoemakers actually built the shoe or boot around the foot. At the Bata Shoe Museum in Toronto you can find leather shoes built in the 1400s that have very high arches, an indication that the shoemakers realized that custom-built corrections were often necessary for their clients, even if they had no technical knowledge of the biomechanics of the foot.

Custom-designed arch supports became very popular in the early 1900s in parts of Europe, and are still commonly sold in regular shoe stores on the Continent. They are manufactured to specific sizes, often with additional frills such as cork or added leather to increase cushioning and comfort. In the 1920s orthotic laboratories sprang up, manufacturing corrective devices they called "arch supports." These were mostly made of leather, but a few manufacturers also used steel in their supports. Most of the work was done by chiropodists, who would take an impression of the foot—for example, by drawing an outline on paper or by making a plaster cast—or, in some cases, using measurements of the foot, followed by a number of fittings during which the leather would be custom-shaped to the patient's foot.

After World War II, laboratories in the

Chapter 2: The Biomechanics of the Foot and Lower Leg

United States began researching and manufacturing custom-made leather orthotics. The word is derived from the Greek *orthos,* which means "straight"—hence, orthotics straighten, or correct, a foot abnormality. They were prescribed by podiatrists and other medical specialists, who would take an impression of the patient's feet and send it to an orthotics laboratory. Most of the impressions were made in plaster, with the patient at rest while his or her feet were cast in a plaster similar to that used for bone fractures; this process provides what we call a *static* measurement procedure. (More recently, static measurement has involved having the patient stand on foam.) Static measurement is still being used today, a situation I have been working hard to remedy with the more accurate *dynamic* computerized system. As we proceed through the book, it will become apparent why dynamic measurement of the foot to reveal its abnormalities is far superior to static measurement.

Orthotics laboratories in the 1970s developed harder, more rigid materials to replace leather—usually different types of plastic, which provided better correction and took up less space in the shoe. Then, as the running craze spread across North America, a need arose for softer orthotics. The laboratories developed softer plastics that provided increased flexibility and shock absorption while maintaining corrective properties. Now well over two hundred compounds are being used for different types of orthotics—graphite being the most

common—and new materials are being developed continuously. Leather inserts are still being sold as alternatives to prescribed orthotics in North American and European shoe stores and specialty shops, but people with definite foot problems will achieve far superior correction with prescribed orthotics.

Different types of orthotics are designed for specific purposes, the most common being for athletic and fashion footwear. It is not unusual for some people to own two or more pairs of orthotics, a slightly bulkier, more cushioned one suitable for wearing when exercising and a thinner one for inserting into tighter-fitting dress shoes.

I now manufacture and prescribe a comprehensive line of orthotics designed to eliminate the majority of foot abnormalities; they have been dynamically measured by a state-of-the-art computerized system. These new orthotics are the result of my lengthy search for the "perfect" correction of biomechanical faults.

By 1990 my colleagues and I had developed a sophisticated computer program for gait analysis using a computerized mat. At the same time I began manufacturing my own orthotics using the digitized printouts, along with the older casting and foam methods. As an experiment, each patient was given one orthotic made from the plaster cast or foam mold and another done by computerization. The results overwhelmingly favored the computerized orthotics. Fully 98 percent of the patients treated much preferred the computer-prescribed orthotic over the other. Corrections were easier to accommodate, the orthotics were more comfortable, and the long-term success rate was much greater.

Aside from a few adults who have difficulty walking at all, or very young children, all my patients are now analyzed using the computerized system, and all those requiring orthotics are given ones designed with the digitized method. Impressive scientific and empirical evidence now suggests that the computerized system can legitimately claim to represent an acceptable standardized methodology for prescribing orthotics.

Over the past three years I have worked very closely on biomechanical foot protocols with leading foot and ankle orthopedic surgeons in the United States to establish medical guidelines for using orthotics for over fifty different foot conditions. This is the first attempt to standardize orthotic foot-therapy care in North America.

Chapter 3

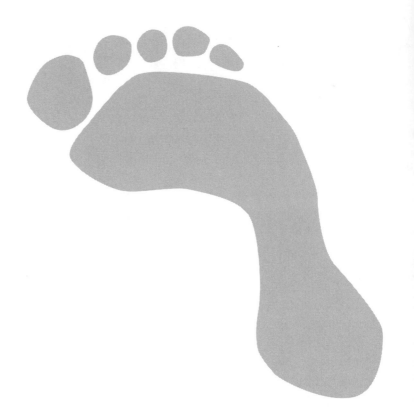

The Bunion and Other Big-Toe Abnormalities

The word *bunion* may derive from the Old English word *bunny*, which meant "a small swelling." But the history of the bunion goes back much further than that. Human beings have been plagued by bunions for thousands of years. If you closely examine some of the earliest Egyptian drawings and writings, you will see and read descriptions of feet obviously deformed by bunions and other big-toe abnormalities.

It wasn't until the 1800s that foot surgeons began experimenting with various surgical remedies for bunions, and rarely with great success. One of their problems was that they had adapted procedures from common types of hand surgery, and people do not normally stand or walk on their hands. Unlike the foot, the hand is not a weight-bearing appendage, so operations that didn't take into consideration the fact that people must constantly put weight on their feet failed miserably. In addition, in those days disinfection of the instruments, the surgeon's hands, the patient's feet, and the bandages was not a priority, and many patients who had foot surgery developed severe infections and other postoperative complications.

Tall Bunion Tales

Contrary to popular belief, bunions are not commonly caused by ill-fitting shoes, although in some cases shoes can worsen the condition. Still, at least one popular medical dictionary states that bunions are "usually caused by ill-fitting shoes." Why, then, do some people living in tropical climes—people who have never worn shoes—develop bunions? Another widely held belief is that the only way to rid yourself of this abnormality is to undergo painful surgery, suffering through a lengthy and uncomfortable recuperation period. I recently saw a young woman with bunions who had put off making her appointment for months because she was afraid I would tell her she required surgery (she didn't). As you will learn in this chapter, many bunions can be treated without surgical intervention, and, fortunately, the surgical horror stories of the past are ancient history. Bunion surgery today is quite sophisticated and far less painful than most people think, and recuperation takes much less time than in the bad old days.

Why Bunions Develop

The medical term for a bunion, *hallux valgus,* can be translated as big, or great, toe (hallux) deforming away from the midline (valgus). What that means in plain English is that there is a deviation in the big-toe joint. In Figure 3.1 you can see how an abnormal big toe deviates from the shape of a normal big toe. Strictly speaking, however, a bunion is a bump, while hallux valgus is a deviation of the big toe, so the two terms are not identical in meaning. But, since they are normally synonymous, I have chosen to use the terms interchangeably, and I trust my purist colleagues will forgive me.

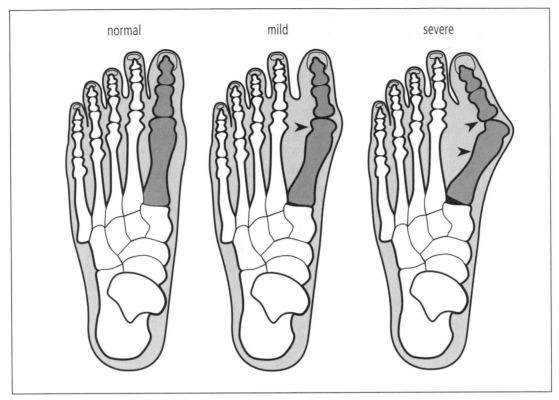

normal   mild   severe

Figure 3.1. Formation of a bunion

Extensive research into the cause and prevention of bunions was encouraged by the frustrating realization over the past few decades that bunions often recur after surgical treatment. Eventually it was discovered that almost all people with bunions pronate abnormally. Using early medical knowledge and theories of cause and effect, the researchers at first deduced that bunions caused abnormal pronation. In other words, a bunion could adversely affect the biomechanics of the foot, which can happen when people change their gait to avoid pain in a sore big toe while walking. However, the researchers quickly realized that the reverse was true: Abnormal pronation causes bunions.

I am often questioned about the heredity factor of bunions. If your grandmother and mother had bunions, will you also succumb to the disorder? The answer is that while a hereditary predisposition may exist, bunions can be prevented if the causes are eliminated. The shape of your foot is obviously determined to a great extent by genetics, just like the color of your hair, eyes, and skin, so a person may be born with a foot that is susceptible to abnormal pronation. However, with proper foot care from the beginning, the incidence of inherited bunions can be reduced. This is particularly true for women who are forefoot pronators; if they regularly wear high heels and are predisposed to developing bunions, they are looking for trouble.

The majority of cases involving bunions actually involve two biomechanical faults: a combination of abnormal subtalar joint pronation and a foot that has an excessively flexible first metatarsal bone. When these two conditions exist, the big-toe joint is called upon to absorb a tremendous amount of weight when the foot is about to push off the ground at the end of the stance phase of the gait cycle—the push-off at the end of the propulsive stage. The reason is that the tendons in the big toe, as they try to counteract the abnormal forces of the pronation and the overly flexible first metatarsal bone, are being asked to stretch and to function in a radically elongated position. This action of the tendons places enormous stress on the big toe, eventually forcing it to deviate to the outside, with the top of the toe pointing toward the baby toe (see Figure 3.1). The big toe exerts pressure on the first metatarsal bone, which is subsequently pulled to the outside. So the *proximal phalanx* (the big bone in the big toe) and the first metatarsal bone are being pulled in opposite directions, like a wishbone. A person with a bunion often winds up with a grotesquely shaped big toe—the result of opposing forces that cannot counterbalance each other without causing a deformity.

There are three basic types of bunion: mild, moderate, and severe. This terminology has nothing to do with the amount of pain involved or the degree of cartilage wear and tear in the big-toe joint. It refers specifically to the degree of deviation of the joint. Some other big-toe joint disorders involve almost no deformity, but produce much more pain than even a severe bunion.

Since the advent of computer and video gait analysis in 1988, we have been able to determine conclusively that most bunions result from an abnormally pronating forefoot. Abnormal pressure placed on the big-toe joint from over-pronation causes a retroactive force on the first metatarsal bone that forces the deviation in the big toe. Over a number of years, this continual retroactive force causes the big toe to point toward the second toe, and it can eventually overlap or underlap the second toe. In order to find nonsurgical resolutions to bunions—not just prevention and treatment of pain—my colleagues have for years been perfecting ways of changing the mechanical forces of the foot by using orthotics. It is my hope that in the near future surgery will become of only historical significance in the treatment of bunions. If computers are able to guide us to corrective and permanent treatment of bunions by using orthotics, surgery may be necessary only in the most severe cases that have been left untreated for years.

One other myth I would like to dispel is about calcium buildup. Clinically, less than 2 percent of the North American population suffers from abnormal calcium levels that affect the big-toe joint; therefore, in most cases, the role of calcium buildup is overrated. Let me state emphatically that bunions are not caused by too much calcium in the body. A bunion is nothing more than a deviation of the great-toe joint resulting from abnormal forces applied to the joint by a biomechanical foot fault. The positions of the first metatarsal and the proximal phalanx clearly change where the bunion is formed, and most of those changes take place where the two bones form the metatarsophalangeal joint. However, this has absolutely nothing to do with too much or too little calcium in the body.

Treating the Bunion

When it comes to treating a bunion, it is logical to assume that the milder the case, the less involved the treatment. Mild, painless bunions that cause no significant discomfort or dysfunction must indeed be treated conservatively (and early) by fitting an orthotic device to eliminate overpronation of the foot, thereby preventing further deviation of the big-toe joint.

Since bunions involve the big-toe joint, and since the joints of the body can become painfully inflamed from irritation (for example, from wearing overly tight shoes), it may occasionally be necessary to treat a mild but angry bunion with an anti-inflammatory drug for a short period of time.

I will have more to say about anti-inflammatory drugs in subsequent chapters, but I would like to point out here that I use them with great discretion, and only to relieve an inflammation, not to cure a particular condition. My main concern with anti-inflammatory drugs, aside from the potentially harmful side effects, is that they do not treat the underlying cause of most of the disorders with which I come into contact. As I continually stress, most of the patients I see have biomechanical faults that will continue to cause discomfort until they have been successfully dealt with. Neither abnormal pronation nor a bunion can be eliminated by taking an anti-inflammatory drug, which helps only in controlling the inflammatory process.

Cortisone injections fall into the same category as oral anti-inflammatory medications. Although they can be quite successful in the treatment of severe joint pain, the benefits do not always outweigh the overall possible risks from injection of a steroid into a joint. Many medical experts strongly believe that cortisone injections into any joint, including the big-toe joint, can accelerate deterioration of the cartilage in that area, thereby negating in the long run any short-term pain relief. It is generally left to the discretion of the physician, after consultation with the patient and evaluation of the risks and benefits of injecting the steroid, to determine whether to proceed with cortisone treatment.

Many people believe that wearing properly fitting shoes will alleviate bunions and the pain associated with them. As you have learned, almost all bunions are caused by poor biomechanics, and not by ill-fitting shoes. However, once a bunion has formed, a shoe with a wide forefoot can alleviate the discomfort associated with a distorted big toe rubbing against tight footwear. But let me stress once again that although people may obtain some relief from their pain, they will still have long-term problems associated with poor biomechanics that the wider shoe cannot address. Of course, tight shoes create nothing but havoc and pain for the bunion sufferer, while properly fitting shoes with a correctly designed orthotic are the ultimate nonsurgical treatment for the bunion.

One more word on shoes: If you have an underlying pronation problem and then wear high heels, which force your foot to abnormally pronate even more, then you are really going to exacerbate your potential for bunion formation.

Aligning the Toe

Unfortunately, many of my bunion patients seek help when they are already past the stage of conservative treatment. For these people, the options are generally limited to surgery or walking barefoot—or in grossly oversized shoes—for the rest of their lives.

Over the past four decades tremendous strides have been made in the surgical resolution of bunions. Previously, the surgeon's repertoire contained two or three procedures for bunion correction. Patients were usually hospitalized, operated on while under a general anesthetic, kept in the hospital for seven to ten days, and fitted with a nonwalking cast for four to eight weeks. Today almost all bunion surgery can be performed on an outpatient basis and under a local anesthetic. A walking cast is placed on the foot, and the patient can convalesce quite comfortably at home. Recovery time will vary with the severity of the condition, but it is normally much faster than with the old surgical techniques. The surgery can be performed by either an orthopedic specialist or a podiatrist. Although the orthopedic surgeon specializing in feet may use slightly different techniques than the podiatrist, the results ought to be the same. I would not hesitate to recommend any number of foot surgeons from both fields.

One other advance in foot surgery is the advent of the scope. Most people are aware of scopes being used in knee, shoulder, and abdominal surgery. In the 1990s scopes were developed to help foot surgeons operate on the joints and other areas of the foot. I believe this will be the way of the future, since the surgeon can clearly view the area that he or she is operating on through a much smaller incision, thereby decreasing the amount of trauma to the surgical site. The surgical instruments used can be passed through the scope so that surgery can be performed in a much more closed environment, without any loss in precision.

Before deciding on the bunion-surgery technique, it is imperative to determine the shape and position of the large big-toe joint. As you can plainly see from Figure 3.1 on page 30, the big-toe bone (proximal phalanx) in a normal foot sits directly ahead of the first metatarsal bone, in an almost straight line when the foot is not in motion. The cartilage of the normal joint is in healthy condition, and the big toe has a range of motion—moving up or down—of at least 45 degrees. This is not the case with a deformed big-toe joint.

The two major concerns with bunions are the position of the metatarsal head vis-à-vis the big-toe joint and the condition of the cartilage in the joint. In many cases of forefoot deformity, a bunion does not actually form in the big toe, but there is so much wear and tear on the big-toe joint that the cartilage erodes and the joint surface flattens. As a result, the range of motion of the big-toe joint diminishes. When this happens, the condition is called *hallux limitus*—not a celestial body, but simply limited motion in the big toe. In severe cases, where there is no motion at all in the big-toe joint, *hallux rigidus* occurs. In some cases, when the cartilage has totally worn out and the joint between the first metatarsal bone and the big-toe bone has become perfectly rigid, the two bones become fused and the joint itself ceases to exist. What we see instead is one long bone, and while the area is now pain-free, there is no longer any joint motion. As a result, the person with such a condition loses a lot of physical mobility. A person suffering from hallux rigidus can experience a great deal of pain until the joint fuses.

Only after the surgeon has fully evaluated the condition of the big-toe joint—by using X rays and manipulation of the toe—can he or she determine precisely which technique best suits the situation. A badly damaged joint will obviously require a totally different approach from that used to treat a mild bunion and a relatively unaffected joint. And, as I have already mentioned, it is entirely possible to have big-toe-joint damage with little or no cartilage remaining, but not have a bunion. In this type of case the surgical procedure changes again.

Hallux Limitus and Hallux Rigidus

As I noted above, hallux limitus and hallux rigidus may or may not accompany bunions, and they can be much more painful. They can respond well to anti-inflammatory medication, physiotherapy, or orthotic devices, but surgical intervention may be required if the discomfort and dysfunction caused by these conditions become unbearable for the patient.

Hallux limitus and hallux rigidus are basically wear-and-tear arthritic disorders, or osteoarthritis. They are examples of painful manifestations of a biomechanical fault. As usual, the culprit is almost always abnormal pronation that results in excess weight being brought to bear on the big-toe joint—weight that the joint was not designed to accept. The pain in the big-toe joint is caused by the wear-and-tear process, which acts to destroy the cushioning cartilage at the ends of the bones. As a result, bone begins to rub against bone—in this case, the head of the metatarsal bone and the end of the big-toe bone—and the irritation produces an inflammation that causes pain. The situation can be compared to throwing sand into a ball-bearing joint in a piece of machinery. The machinery cannot run smoothly with the foreign objects grinding on its moving parts.

This pain in the big-toe joint is often mistaken for gout or some other systemic arthritis-type disease. But in 99 percent of the cases, the problem is osteoarthritis. It pains me that I still occasionally see patients who are being treated with medication for gout, even though all the blood tests for the disease were negative. I shall have much more to say about gout in Chapter 10; although it affects the big-toe joint, it belongs in a discussion of systemic diseases that affect the foot.

It is possible to treat hallux limitus and hallux rigidus nonsurgically, as we would treat a mild bunion, if the diagnosis is made early enough, before severe deterioration of the joint has taken place. However, if deterioration of the joint is extensive and the pain is severe, surgical intervention must be considered, particu-

larly for hallux rigidus. Three quite successful open surgery procedures are used for repair of the big-toe joint.

One of the treatments we practiced in the seventies and eighties was Silastic joint replacement for the big-toe joint. Unfortunately, as most people learned in the early 1990s, silicone breast implants have been linked to potentially serious health problems in patients who have received them. Silastic implants are a close cousin to silicone implants, and we found in the 1990s that a small number of people may have developed minor bone reactions to them.

Postoperative Care

Just because bunion surgery and other big-toe surgery no longer require a hospital stay, the patient must not be lulled into believing that the toe will miraculously recover all by itself. Patients must follow numerous rules. Aerobics, running, and dancing are out! Since the recovery routine varies with the severity of the operation, I will not attempt to go into great detail about what to do and what not to do. What I want to stress here and throughout the book is the importance of communicating with the surgeon and understanding fully what you must do following surgery to ensure a rapid, trouble-free recovery. As you might suspect, the more complicated the surgery is, the lengthier the recuperation period. In any event, you will not be able to run a marathon immediately following the operation. On the other hand, if you follow the surgeon's instructions, you should be relatively free of discomfort after the operation, and you ought to be able to resume normal physical activities in a matter of weeks.

A Final Word Before Leaving the Joint

Regardless of the condition of the big toe and its need for surgery, to prevent renewed deterioration and/or deviation of the big-toe joint, the biomechanical fault causing the problem must be eliminated with a proper orthotic device. Otherwise, no matter how much you play around with the joint, the problems will continue. The sole exception is when the cause of the trouble is a systemic disorder.

I want to emphasize the importance of good doctor–patient communication. As a patient, you must know precisely what bunion or other big-toe surgery will do for you, and the doctor must be aware of your expectations. A patient who does not get what he or she bargained for will not be happy.

Patients often believe that their arthritis will be totally relieved following surgery. Although the doctor has not said so, many patients also believe that the big toe will be perfectly normal again after the surgery. Patients regularly fail to ask about potential side effects of their surgery. Either they do not suspect that there will be any, or they don't want to know, as long as the pain is eliminated. The doctor might forget to tell the patient about the side effects of an operation that involves fusion of the big-toe joint, or might decide that the patient will not understand or will not want to know. Instead of the expected painless big toe with a normal range of motion, the patient winds up with a painless but fused big toe that cannot be manipulated. He or she has unwittingly sacrificed a degree of mobility for pain relief and may feel that the operation was less than totally successful. On the other hand, the surgeon believes that the operation was a total success, since it accomplished precisely what he or she set out to do: to completely eliminate the patient's pain.

The moral of this story is, if you are the patient, do not hesitate to ask all the questions that come to mind. If you are the doctor, make sure that the patient fully understands the nature of the condition, the treatment involved, and the potential side effects of that treatment. Such communication will save a lot of misery on both sides.

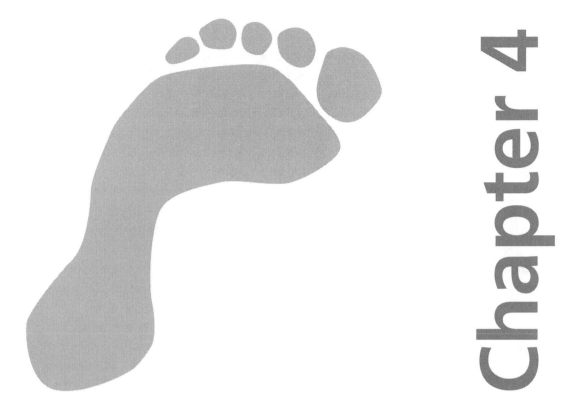

Problems of
the Forefoot

Chapter 4: Problems of the Forefoot

As you will remember from Chapter 1, the forefoot is composed of five metatarsal bones; two phalanges (phalanx bones) in the great toe and three phalanges in the other toes; two sesamoid bones under the first metatarsal; joints; soft tissue such as muscles, tendons, ligaments, and other connective tissue; nerves; and veins, arteries, and smaller blood vessels that provide the area with a steady supply of fresh nutrients.

The forefoot is the workhorse of the foot, because it is in contact with the ground 75 percent of the time during the stance phase of the gait cycle (that is, when you are in stride). Therefore it receives most of the pounding to which the foot is subjected when a person is walking, running, or doing other stressful things in an upright position.

Unlike the rearfoot and the midfoot, which have a few, very solid bone structures, the forefoot has twenty-one bones that work together intricately to help propel the leg forward. So it is not surprising that more can go wrong with the forefoot than with the rest of the foot, particularly as weight distribution on the bottom of the foot is normally far greater at the front. Considering the odds against the forefoot, it is surprising that less than 5 percent of the North American population will ever break a toe, and less than one percent will ever fracture a metatarsal bone. This is amazing, considering what klutzes some of us are and the willingness of many of us to wear improper shoes.

The most common problems involving the forefoot are calluses and corns, which we will deal with in subsequent chapters. However, other disorders affecting the forefoot are quite interesting—and distressing—and we will discuss them here. Most of these problems involve inflammations of tendons, ligaments, joints, and nerves, but a few concern fractures of the many bones in the forefoot.

In a typical conversation about foot pain between a doctor and a patient, the doctor might tell the patient that the problem is *metatarsalgia*. The patient becomes anxious because the word sounds ominous. But all metatarsalgia means is pain in the area of the metatarsal bones in the forefoot. In essence, the doctor is merely agreeing with the patient that he or she has a sore forefoot.

Now, if you went to a doctor and told him that you had a stomachache, and were informed after a cursory examination that you had a sore stomach, would you be satisfied with the diagnosis? I should hope not, especially if the doctor were to tell you that it was untreatable or that an operation ought to be performed to investigate. Well, the same applies to the forefoot. Never settle for a diagnosis of metatarsalgia without a full explanation, because it is merely a catch-all term. If a doctor tells you that your foot pain will magically disappear on its own, that you will have to learn to live with it, or that the foot ought to be dissected to better evaluate the situation, run out of the office as fast as you can—if you can still run—in search of another opinion.

The possible reasons for metatarsalgia may involve inflammation and/or fractures of a bone, as well as a whole host of soft-tissue problems, and treatment must obviously vary with the disorder. Keep in mind that forefoot pain is almost never indicative of a major disease, and the cause of the pain is rarely terribly difficult to treat.

A Metatarsal Headache

When a patient complains of pain in the metatarsal area, one of the problems a foot specialist faces is properly diagnosing the condition. Many disorders have symptoms that mimic each other, and it takes an expert to determine the actual cause of the discomfort. Let us examine one of the most common causes of visits to my office: metatarsal-head pain.

One of the causes of metatarsal-head pain is a *plantar-flexed* metatarsal bone (see Figure 2.3 on page 21 and Figure 6.1 on page 65) that does not drop down as it should when you walk; rather, it is always down. The primary reason it cannot move back up is wear and tear at the midtarsal joint. It sits lower than the other metatarsal heads, which naturally rise and drop during the normal gait cycle. As a result, the plantar-flexed metatarsal bone is always bearing shock by itself, and directly on the end of its head. The problem is exacerbated by ill-fitting shoes, particularly those with very thin soles, which have little cush-

ioning for absorbing shock during walking or running. The shock often winds up being absorbed by the metatarsal heads. By the time metatarsal-head pain has begun, even comfortable, shock-absorbing shoes will probably be of little help. Once the metatarsal head has become inflamed, only total elimination of the irritation will calm the area.

The heads of the metatarsal bones form *metatarso-phalangeal joints* with the proximal phalanges (the largest bones in the toes). A plantar flexion will cause irritation at the offending joint that can take the form of either capsulitis or synovitis. A *capsule* is the lining on the outside of a joint; a *synovium* is the lining on the inside of a joint. Hence we use the terms *capsulitis* and *synovitis* to describe inflammations of these linings. In this case, the inflammation is of the linings of the metatarso-phalangeal joint.

The major symptom of these types of inflammation is a sensation like a bad bruise in the troubled area, almost as if the sufferer had stepped on a stone. Unfortunately, this symptom is somewhat similar to that of a neuroma (a nerve condition discussed later in this chapter), because the inflamed area is very close to the *interspace* through which the nerve passes. Victims of this condition will often complain that they hurt much more when they are off their feet, and many awaken with terrible pain in the affected area. The reason for this is swelling that builds up at the inflamed site when the foot is at rest. When the person is walking, the swelling is diffused by the foot's constantly striking the ground, and therefore rarely builds up in one area to the point where the inflammation severely affects the nerves. At night, when there is no pressure on the foot, the swelling concentrates at the area of the plantar flexion and eventually inflames the nerves to such an extent that excruciating pain is experienced.

Our old friend abnormal pronation is also a prime cause of metatarsal-head pain. Unlike plantar flexion, however, it does not involve just one faulty metatarsal bone; the biomechanical fault is spread widely across the entire foot.

As you now know, when a foot pronates, the weight on the foot moves across the metatarsal heads from the baby toe over to the big toe. Each metatarsal head is subjected to weight at slightly different times, rather than all together with the others. Therefore, when you are walking or running, for a brief interval each head is absorbing 100 percent of the weight of your body. That places tremendous stress on each metatarsal head with every step.

You will also recall that when a foot pronates, it rolls from the outside in. Something has to stop that roll; otherwise, if you overpronated severely you would walk very strangely, for you would be constantly turning or twisting your foot as you completed each step. What happens is that the big toe provides support to break the roll, and the foot widens and forces the big toe to angle inward. The result is that the first and sec-ond metatarsal heads act together to absorb enough force to halt the roll. If a person overpronates significantly, the second metatarsal head receives a large amount of the abnormal force and becomes inflamed; the big toe angles further inward, and eventually the detour causes a bunion.

This action can produce metatarsal-head pain in the second metatarsal bone. The discomfort is quite similar in symptoms to pain induced by plantar flexion, and therefore is also difficult to distinguish from neuroma-induced pain. To complicate matters even further, it is possible, though uncommon, to suffer from both a neuroma and metatarsal-head pain at the same time. The metatarsal heads are so close to the nerves passing through the interspaces that one inflammation can trigger another. For example, a metatarsal head that is inflamed will cause swelling around the nerve. This swelling may eventually constrict the space through which the nerve must pass, thereby setting up the possible development of a neuroma. In this situation, the symptoms will mimic those of both a neural and a metatarsal-head problem, which will complicate both diagnosis and treatment of the conditions, as you can imagine.

There has been much speculation as to which comes first, the metatarsal-head disorder or the neuroma. In my opinion, metatarsal-head inflammation will usually result in the development of nerve inflammation, although the reverse is definitely possible.

I have had excellent success over the years in diagnosing these disorders and determining which of the two conditions exists. In the hands of a well-trained practitioner, new diagnostic ultrasound machines have now made it possible to view this area of soft-tissue inflammation. My basic technique for establishing the existence of metatarsal-head pain is by *palpating* (using my hands and fingertips to probe the affected area) directly over the metatarsal head. If this produces pain, I can be reasonably secure in my diagnosis, particularly if the tests for a neuroma are negative. (I will describe later how I test for nerve inflammation.)

Treating Metatarsal Pain

How do we treat metatarsal pain caused by a biomechanical fault in the foot? You guessed it: with orthotics to correct the fault and, on rare occasions when necessary, an injected or oral anti-inflammatory drug, along with ultrasound treatment or laser therapy to alleviate the inflammation if it is severe. Although the problem is often one of abnormal shock-absorption stress on the metatarsal heads, simple shock-absorption pads cannot correct the metatarsal-head weight-distribution problem. I used to believe that the orthotics might always have to be worn since, once a person is fully grown, metatarsal problems may not cure themselves. However, with the introduction of computerized gait analysis we now believe that plantar-flexed

metatarsal-head problems may be fixable over time by using orthotics that are based on in-shoe computer analysis. Our initial observations indicate that complete recovery can take place over a few years, at which time orthotics may no longer be required. As we do follow-up examinations of our patients, we expect these findings to be confirmed.

Surgery is a last resort for treatment of metatarsal-head pain. However, if the metatarsal head is severely dropped down and is causing all sorts of mischief, such as painful calluses under the head, a metatarsal *osteotomy* may be the only way to permanently correct the problem. This procedure involves breaking the metatarsal bone and repositioning it to allow for normal metatarsal-head function. It is not as gruesome as it sounds, and can produce excellent results with a minimum of discomfort during the healing stage, providing that postoperative care instructions are followed.

Of course, there can be problems with an osteotomy, whether it involves metatarsal bones or any other bones in the body. The major concern is failure of the bones broken during the surgical procedure to reunite. In normal circumstances, the severed ends of the bone will rejoin naturally over a period of time, and you will eventually have one whole bone again—one that is biomechanically normal and that will not place undue stress on the metatarsal head.

The second problem that may occur

with osteotomy of a metatarsal bone is that the floating end of the bone may move to an abnormally high position and cause a problem with an adjacent metatarsal bone. If, for example, the floating piece of the second metatarsal bone sits so high that its head no longer supports any weight, the third metatarsal head will then be subjected to the brunt of the body weight distributed in that area when the person is in stride. It will become inflamed because of the added weight it must bear, until it too eventually requires medical treatment— perhaps an osteotomy of its own. This used to happen about 20 percent of the time after an osteotomy of a metatarsal bone. However, by fixing the induced fracture with a pin or surgical screw, the sur-

geon can now position the fracture site at the angle that best suits its bony neighbors.

A Bad Case of Nerves

A *neuroma* is a benign tumor of a nerve caused by abnormal growth of nerve cells in response to an irritation. Let me emphasize that a neuroma in the forefoot is never more than a simple irritated pinched nerve that causes pain because of constant compression and irritation, either between metatarsal heads or at the base of the proximal phalanges (the largest bones in the toes). You can see the area where neuromas are most likely to occur in Figure 4.1.

A neuroma may develop when poor biomechanical function of the foot causes

Figure 4.1. Metatarsal bones and their problems

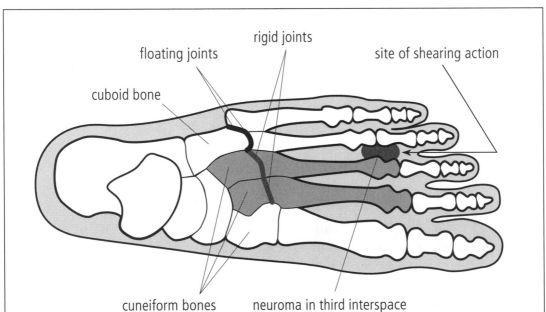

chronic irritation of a nerve, thereby triggering the growth of additional nerve cells. The extra nerve tissue is nature's way of trying to protect the nerve from further irritation, but, because a vicious cycle develops, the opposite occurs. That extra nerve tissue takes up space and forces further irritation because it is now even closer to the offending bone structure. Then, as the nerve becomes further inflamed, it develops more tissue to protect its core and thus further compresses the space through which it must pass. This merry-go-round continues until the owner of the foot seeks medical attention because the discomfort has become too extreme to ignore.

The second most likely cause of a neuroma, which often acts in conjunction with the first, is wearing ill-fitting shoes that squeeze the forefoot and also force it to accept almost all of the body's weight during walking or running. The worst culprits are ladies' high-heeled shoes. The third possible cause of a neuroma is swelling of the foot, for whatever reason, which reduces the space through which the nerves must pass. The fourth, and least common, cause is an abnormal bony structure or growth that pinches the nerve as it tries to pass through the areas normally reserved for its passage.

Aside from the causes I have mentioned, two theories attempt to explain more clinically the origin of a neuroma. The first theory is that there is a difference between the way the second and third metatarsal bones articulate (meet to form a joint) with the cuneiform bones behind them, and the way the fourth and fifth metatarsal bones articulate with the cuboid bone behind them (see Figure 4.1). The second and third metatarsal bones form a basically rigid joint with their respective cuneiform bones; the fourth and fifth metatarsal bones form a movable joint with the cuboid bone. In a sense, the fourth and fifth metatarsals "float," and the action of the fourth, in contrast to the rigid third metatarsal, results in a shearing effect at the interspace between the third and fourth metatarsals. When the fourth metatarsal bone shears down, it cuts at the space through which the nerve passes. Naturally, the nerve may then become irritated and a neuroma may develop.

To understand the second theory, you have to imagine the path of the *posterior tibial nerve,* which runs down the back of the leg and splits into the *medial* and *lateral plantar nerves* once it enters the foot itself. The medial nerve runs along the bottom of the foot to the big-toe side, while the lateral nerve travels along the bottom of the foot to the baby-toe side.

As it approaches the area of the metatarsal bones, the medial plantar nerve branches out, one twig passing through the first interspace between the toes, the next one through the second interspace, and the third through the third interspace. The lateral plantar nerve branches into two twigs—one passing through the third interspace, the other through the fourth. If you have been counting, you realize that two separate tiny nerves run through the third interspace. That double thickness of nerve explains the greater frequency of neuromas at the third interspace. Whoever designed the foot apparently goofed by not compensating adequately for the extra amount of nerve tissue in that area.

The most common site of a forefoot neuroma is at the third interspace, between the third and fourth toes (see Figure 4.1). It was first identified by Dr. Dudley Morton, an early pioneer of research into foot disorders—hence the name *Morton's neuroma*. In descending order of occurrence are neuromas of the second interspace, the first, and the fourth.

The symptoms of a forefoot neuroma generally vary from patient to patient and can range from mild to severe. The most common symptom is a burning sensation in the area of the neuroma-affected toes. Some patients will experience a popping or dislocating sensation in the interspace involved. Many people with the disorder also feel a generalized ache or pain in the offending interspace, sometimes accompanied by the unpleasant sensation of a hot knife cutting through the bottom of the foot. The discomfort will inevitably be exacerbated by wearing shoes that are too tight, particularly those with high heels that force extra weight onto the forefoot.

One of the tests I use to determine the presence of a neuroma is *Mulder's sign,* named after the doctor who invented the diagnostic procedure. I place my right thumb under the involved interspace and use the left hand to squeeze together the metatarsal heads. If a neuroma is there, it will create a sharp, popping sensation, and the patient will probably curse loudly, since the painful symptoms of the disorder will be produced in spades by the squeezing. The bigger the pop, the larger the neuroma. This test is about 85 percent accurate in distinguishing neuromas from metatarsal-head pain.

Treating Nervous Breakdown of the Foot

Unfortunately I cannot give you a 100 percent guarantee when it comes to treatment of a neuroma. The best I can cite is a 75 percent success rate, regardless of the cause or the treatment method.

Treatment is based on the cause of the disorder. If the problem has been caused primarily by improper footwear, the obvious thing to do first is to change shoes—permanently. At the same time, if the neuroma is causing the patient a lot of discomfort, I may opt to inject cortisone with an anesthetic into the area around the inflamed nerve. Relief will occur in about 30 percent of cases, although initially (for a couple of days) the discomfort may actually increase, because the injection can itself irritate the nerve.

In most neuroma cases, computer gait analysis is very helpful in determining the cause(s) of the neuroma. If the problem is caused by a biomechanical fault, orthotics based on that analysis will work up to 80 percent of the time.

If the neuroma does not respond well to the above treatments and is severe enough to drastically restrict the patient's regular activities, I may consider surgery. However, I would choose this path only if the patient's quality of life has become abysmal because of the discomfort. I am most reluctant to perform nerve surgery, because it is tricky and does not always produce the desired effect. Surgery for a severely inflamed neuroma involves removal of the affected portion of the nerve. It can be done in a doctor's office under a local anesthetic, and it takes about half an hour to perform. The patient can walk immediately and ought to be completely recovered after six to eight weeks. During the recovery period, the discomfort should be only a tiny fraction of what it was before the neuroma was removed.

March Break: The Stress Fracture

In the United States Marine Corps it used to be common to test the mettle of new recruits by sending them out on twenty-mile runs after only a short period of boot-camp training. To make the test a bit more sadistic, the recruits were forced to wear army boots rather than running shoes. You try running twenty miles in heavy boots when you're out of shape! Subsequently, about 5 percent of the recruits were found to have so-called march fractures of a metatarsal bone, caused by the stress of running in abnormal footwear. We are familiar with the condition by its more common name, *stress fracture*. The metatarsal bone most likely to be involved is the second (50 percent of the time), next is the third (25 percent), and the other 25 percent of cases involve the fourth metatarsal. I have never seen a stress fracture of either the first or the fifth metatarsal bone.

A stress fracture of a bone is caused by excessive, often continuous, pressure on a part of the bone for a given time, particularly over a lengthy period. It is fairly common, medically speaking, in metatarsal bones, but can also occur in most of the bones of the foot and lower leg. Novice Marines are not the only people susceptible to the condition. It also affects a lot of runners who overstress one part of their feet, aerobic exercisers who partake to excess, and women who walk long distances in high-heeled shoes that place extra pressure on the forefoot. A metatarsal bone can also sustain a stress fracture when the foot attempts to deal naturally with a plantar-flexion problem. Once that plantar-flexed metatarsal has broken on its own, it will be quite sore, but weight distribution on the metatarsal heads should become fairly normal.

You might imagine that a fracture would show up clearly enough on an X ray, but such is not the case with a stress fracture—unless it is quite severe—until about four to six weeks have elapsed from the time of the break. When it does show up on an X ray, what is seen is the bone-healing callus that forms around fractured bone ends and is essential for healthy reuniting of the ends of the bone.

So if a stress fracture does not show up on an X ray, how is it diagnosed? One way is to palpate the shaft of the metatarsal bone. If pressing on the offending part of the bone produces pain, you become suspicious. Also, if a break has occurred, the area on top of the metatarsal bone will be quite swollen. In some instances where diagnosis is difficult, a *bone scan* is done, in which radioactive dye is painlessly injected into the bloodstream. If the test shows a "hot spot" where a break is suspected, generally the diagnosis is confirmed.

Treatment of Stress Fractures

A foot-bone fracture, whether of the stress variety or caused by a severe traumatic incident, will normally heal on its own. Unlike other fractured bones in the body, the metatarsals are not thrown out of alignment by a stress fracture. Therefore, a cast is not required to immobilize the mending bone in the proper position. This fact makes a stress fracture easier to live with during the recovery period. However, the damaged bone must not be stressed further by activities that put excessive pressure on the forefoot—that is, the type of activity that caused the fracture in the first

place. These types of activities include running, playing racket sports, and similar athletic endeavors. Also, during the recovery period women must avoid wearing high-heeled shoes that put extra stress on the forefoot. Comfortable running shoes are the perfect footwear for the normal three-week recovery period.

Ultrasound treatment is definitely *not* recommended for a stress fracture. Ultrasound waves seem to interfere with the natural healing process of broken bones. A few patients have described to me the suffering they endured from pain produced by wrongly prescribed ultrasound treatment. The problem is not with uneducated therapists, but rather with an initial misdiagnosis of the problem. Stress fractures, as I mentioned above, can easily be mistaken for other metatarsal disorders.

Finally, use a bit of common sense. If you have been diagnosed as having a metatarsal stress fracture, you will have to exercise a bit of patience until the break has healed on its own. If you try to push yourself—for example, by running too soon or wearing high heels before the break has healed—you will compound your suffering and push back the date of your recovery by a few weeks.

The Sesamoid Bones

Two bones, the *sesamoids,* sit under the first metatarsal bone at the big-toe joint (see Figure 1.1, on page 7). These sesame seed–shaped bones seem to have little function vis-à-vis the biomechanics of the foot. According to evolutionary theory, they are thought to be left over from our ancestors, who may have spent more time on all fours than most of us do nowadays.

Although the sesamoid bones have minimal effect on the biomechanics of the human foot—unless they fracture or become an area of inflammation—the same is not true for horses. Sesamoid fractures are not uncommon in racehorses because of the pounding the equine hoof takes while the horse is running, and when that unfortunate break occurs, the horse sometimes has to be destroyed. That is not to say that humans are able to avoid sesamoid problems, but the solution is considerably less drastic.

Sesamoid bones can fracture, unfortunately, and the soft tissue around the bones can become painfully inflamed. The reason for this is twofold. First, the sesamoid bones sit very close to the surface of the foot. Second, in the case of a plantar-flexed first metatarsal bone, they are in direct contact with the ground. This condition is called a *forefoot valgus* deformity (see Figure 2.3, on page 21). While the deformity itself does not cause discomfort or dysfunction, it does expose the sesamoid bones to undue stress that can lead to problems in the area.

Sesamoiditis is an inflammation of the area under the first metatarsal head of the big-toe joint. It can be caused by a forefoot valgus deformity that exposes the sesamoids, by an activity that places extra pres-

sure on the area, or by trauma. For example, a person with a forefoot valgus deformity who plays a racket sport, which requires a lot of stop-and-start running and excessive pressures on a specific part of the foot, could be irritating their sesamoids. The same holds true for a woman with such a deformity who wears high-heeled shoes that put extra pressure on the first metatarso-phalangeal joint (MPJ) and the sesamoid bones beneath. The inflammation can occur right under the sesamoid bone or between it and the metatarsal bone above it. When the latter happens, the cartilage between the two bones becomes irritated, and after a few years it can degenerate to the point where bone is left rubbing directly against bone.

How do you know if you are suffering from sesamoiditis? If, when the area is palpated, you have a considerable amount of pain and tenderness on the bottom of the foot under the big-toe joint, you are a good candidate for a diagnosis of sesamoiditis. The discomfort is akin to that of capsulitis or synovitis of the MPJ, and can be exacerbated by wearing improper footwear, such as high-heeled shoes that put undue pressure on the forefoot when the sufferer is walking. The pain may begin gradually and might take a while to reach potentially unbearable levels. In some cases, numbness may also be felt in the affected area because of the proximity of the *proper digital nerve,* which may itself become inflamed because of irritation caused by the sesamoiditis. It is often difficult to determine whether the problem is sesamoiditis or a stress fracture of a sesamoid bone. Generally there is much more swelling if a bone is broken, and the onset of pain after the break is rapid and intense.

The treatment of sesamoiditis depends in large part on the cause of the disorder. If the problem originated from a forefoot valgus deformity, the use of orthotics to correct the abnormality is advised. This treatment by itself ought to provide quick relief to the area, without the need for drugs or other therapy. If the condition resulted from a trauma such as a sports injury, ultrasound and ice ought to quiet down the area, and the inflammation will clear up on its own. If the sesamoiditis is chronic, cortisone injections seem to work quite well, but these should only be considered as a last resort.

The sesamoids can fracture if exposed to trauma or overstress. When this happens, the patient experiences pain in the area of the fracture. The fracture will show up on X rays, but there is nonetheless a problem with diagnosis. About a fifth of all people have a *bipartite* (split in two) sesamoid bone from birth. This congenital condition is harmless and painless, but when X rays are taken of the area, the bipartite bone can be mistaken for a fractured single bone. To clear up the dilemma, it may be necessary to do a bone scan to determine whether or not the sesamoid has actually been fractured. The appearance of a hot spot on the scan will tell the tale.

Treatment of a fractured sesamoid, short of shooting the patient, is not easy. The problem is the poor supply of blood to the area, combined with the constant pounding on that part of the foot caused by walking or running. Once broken, a sesamoid bone will usually remain bipartite, but the pain should eventually subside and disappear.

If the pain persists to the point that it affects the patient's quality of life, a surgical approach should definitely be considered. The surgery involves removal of the offending parts of the bone, but it is not a major procedure. In fact, it can be done under local anesthetic on an outpatient basis, and the patient will be quite comfortable and walking right after the operation. Recovery time depends on the patient's willingness to let the area heal naturally, with as little stress on it as possible, until no discomfort is experienced during normal activities.

The Midfoot and the Baby Toe

I have discussed various conditions that can affect various parts of the foot, but I have said almost nothing (and will continue to say very little) about the midfoot. Look back at Figure 1.1 (page 7) to refresh your memory. It will remind you that the midfoot has five bones: the navicular, three cuneiforms, and the cuboid. These bones articulate with the metatarsals in the forefoot and the calcaneus (heel bone) in the rearfoot, so the midtarsal joint plays a role in the biomechanical function of the foot.

There is very little movement in the midtarsal joint, so a disorder arising there is far more unlikely than in other parts of the foot. The bones of the midfoot are also very thick, almost cube-shaped, and therefore quite able to withstand punishment unless severely traumatized by some crushing accident. In my years of practice I have seen only one fractured cuboid bone, and that belonged to a weightlifter who was either careless or overly optimistic and dropped a weight on his foot.

Certain biomechanical abnormalities, however, place undue stress on the midtarsal joint. As a result, some early wear and tear can arise and cause mild abnormal degeneration—which could later cause osteoarthritis. But in most cases the condition never becomes very dramatic, and a person prone to some midfoot wear and tear will hardly notice any symptoms.

The midfoot can be affected by certain neuromuscular disorders that can cause loss of sensitivity in the area and, therefore, an inability to control movement of the foot. These conditions can also cause significant degenerative changes in the midtarsal joint. However, I have seen very few people with such neuromuscular diseases, so rather than worry you with details about them, I prefer to tell you that the chances of your being hit by one are quite remote.

I have neglected the fifth, or baby, toe. Other than its being injured or affected by corns, the only thing that can go wrong with it is a *bunionette*—also known as a baby bunion, a tailor's bunion, or a fifth metatarsal-head bunion.

Baby-toe bunions are similar to their big-toe brothers and can be caused by two biomechanical foot faults. The first is usually congenital and occurs when the angle between the fourth and the fifth metatarsal bones is more than 20 degrees. Not everyone who has this abnormality will get a bunionette, but the odds increase when the angle is wider, particularly when the second biomechanical problem also occurs: a plantar-flexed fifth metatarsal. In response to the extra pressure applied to the area because the metatarsal head is never raised, the bone moves laterally away from the midpoint of the foot in an attempt to distribute weight more evenly. In response to the irritation in the area, a bump eventually appears on the outside of the toe at the fifth metatarsal head. This bump corresponds to a bunion on the big toe, but is tinier. Hence, the term bunionette or baby bunion.

Because of the congenital nature of the problem, it is quite difficult to prevent formation of a bunionette. Once the irritation has become a real pain to the victim, the only recourse is usually surgery. The surgery involves two procedures: an *exostectomy,* or removal of the bump on the toe, followed by an osteotomy to realign the metatarsal bone. Most of the time this surgery is successful, whether done "open" or by using a minimal-incision surgery (MIS) technique, and the patient's metatarsal returns to normal after a four- to six-week recovery period.

The Fifth Metatarsal

Another area that is often overlooked in discussions of foot problems is the base of the fifth metatarsal bone. Moderately to severely turning an ankle inward *(lateral inversion)* can cause an *avulsion fracture* of the base of this bone. This occurs because of the dramatic force put on the bone, and is often overlooked by doctors examining and X-raying a suspected ankle fracture or similar type of injury.

The reason the fracture can be so easily overlooked is that the ankle bone (talus) is so close to the base of the fifth metatarsal bone, and swelling in the area can be confused with a reaction to the ankle injury. The clinician must examine the area carefully to avoid making a mistake. If X rays confirm a fifth metatarsal bone fractured at its base, the treatment is much the same as it would be for a stress fracture of any other metatarsal bone. The break will heal by itself over a period of weeks without the foot having to be put in a cast or otherwise treated, but the victim of the injury will have to be careful during the recovery time to avoid placing undue stress on the area.

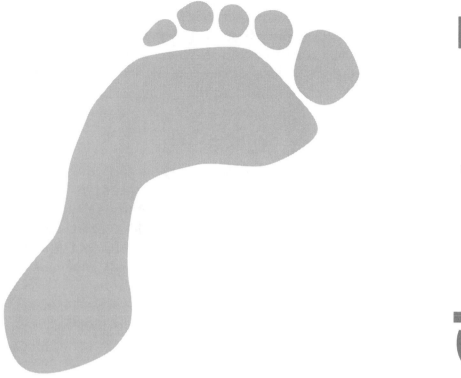

Chapter 5

Hammer Toes
and Corns

Hammer toes and corns are conditions that often go together. I will explain to you shortly why this is so, but first let me tell you a little about corns, because people are often misinformed about them.

A Kernel of Truth

The word *corn*, as it applies to a protrusion on the skin, has absolutely nothing to do with the plant that sprouts ears. It comes from the Latin word *cornu*, which literally means "horn." At some time during the course of European history, a comparison was made between a thickened area of skin on or between the toes and a horny protuberance.

In medicalese, a corn is called a *heloma*, and by definition it is a protrusion on the top or side of a toe. About two-thirds of all corns occur on the top of the toe and develop in response to contraction of the offending digit. The toe may have been bent because of a biomechanical foot fault or, occasionally, because of improperly fitting shoes. A third of all corns are so-called "soft" or "wet" corns, and they occur on the sides of the toes. They are caused primarily by biomechanical faults.

Many people confuse corns and calluses. The dif-ference between the two is that a callus appears only on the bottom of the foot. However, both are thickened areas of skin, and both are caused primarily by biomechanical foot faults.

Hammer Toe

One of the primary causes of corns on the top of the toe is *hammer toe*. As you can see in Figure 5.1, a hammer toe is abnormally contracted and bent. This situation develops over a period of years and finally reaches a point at which it becomes obvious—and painful. Unfortunately, a person does not normally notice its development until the area begins to hurt, likely making fitting into a pair of shoes a very painful experience.

Figure 5.1. Hammer toe

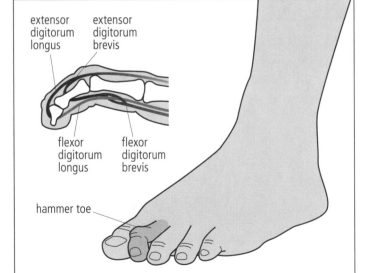

extensor digitorum longus

extensor digitorum brevis

flexor digitorum longus

flexor digitorum brevis

hammer toe

Speaking of shoes, the common belief is that tight and other poorly fitting shoes are the primary causes of hammer toes. I beg to differ. As with bunions, one has only to examine the feet of African Bushmen who have never worn shoes to discover that many of them also have hammer toes.

So if shoes are not normally to blame for the development of hammer toes, what is? As you may have suspected, the culprit is generally our old nemesis, the biomechanical fault. But this time we have to look at the muscles and tendons on top of and below the toe bones to discover how they can cause the toe to form the shape of a hammer. If you examine Figure 5.1, you will see exactly where these muscles and tendons are located.

We are going to talk here about flexor and extensor muscles, so let me explain briefly the difference between the two. *Flexor muscles* cause the bending (flexing) movements of a limb or other body part; *extensor muscles,* on the other hand, cause a straightening (extending) movement.

The muscles on the tops of the toes, with the exception of the big toe, are called the *extensor digitorum longus* and the *extensor digitorum brevis*. Those on the underside of these four toes are called the *flexor digitorum longus* and the *flexor digitorum brevis*. The corresponding muscles on the big toe are the *extensor hallucis longus,* the *extensor hallucis brevis,* the *flexor hallucis longus,* and the *flexor hallucis brevis*. (I hope you memorize all these, be-

cause there is a test at the end of this chapter!) Together, these muscles control the movements of each toe. When something happens to cause at least one of the muscles to malfunction, the biomechanics of the toe involved will also become abnormal. The most common result is a hammer toe, and once a hammer toe develops, a corn cannot be far behind.

All the toes, with the exception of the big toe, have three bones, so there are two interphalangeal joints in each of the four lesser toes (see Figure 1.1, on page 7). When we refer to hammer toes, we mean a contracture of the *proximal* joint, which is farther from the tip of the toe. When we talk about *mallet toes,* which look similar to hammer toes, we are referring to the *distal* joint, closer to the tip of the toe. When both interphalangeal joints are contracted, the condition is called a *claw toe*. However, some health-care professionals use the terms interchangeably. Rather than confuse the issue, I will refer primarily to hammer toe, which is the most commonly used name for this contracture condition. (Actually, a mallet toe on the distal interphalangeal joint is different from a contracture on the proximal joint. It can be brought on by tight shoes and/or tight hosiery to a far greater extent than a hammer toe can be, even though the primary cause of both contractures is still biomechanical. However, the symptoms, diagnosis, and treatment for both are basically identical.)

If we examine the biomechanics of the

foot as they relate to the toes, we can understand how hammer toes develop. When the subtalar joint pronates abnormally, it creates excessive mobility in the forefoot—specifically in the metatarsophalangeal joints. As with bunions, one abnormally positioned bone forces another to deviate as well. A plantar-flexed metatarsal head (which sits closer to the ground than the other metatarsal heads) will force the flexor digitorum longus (FDL) and flexor digitorum brevis tendons on the bottom of the toes to tighten, as the corresponding muscles try to compensate for the abnormality and keep the metatarsal and toe bones aligned properly. When the muscles are pulled tight, the tendons at the ends of the muscles are stretched to their limits. You will recall from our chapter on the anatomy of the foot that tendons are under stress whenever muscles are stretched beyond their limits. When the FDL muscles and their tendons are overstressed, the situation is similar to a rope attached to the end of a fixed flexible tube and passing through it. If the free end of the rope is pulled tight, the tube begins to bend in or near the middle and to bunch up. This is what happens with a toe that has overstressed muscles and tendons, and the end result is a hammer-shaped toe (see Figure 5.1).

Although a large number of the patients with hammer toes that I see acquired the syndrome through a biomechanical fault, there are other causes as well. Most of them do indeed result from constantly wearing shoes that do not fit properly. What usually happens is that a shoe that is too short, narrow, or shallow for the foot places constant abnormal pressure on the toes by causing them to contract or twist. Women who wear shoes with four-inch spike heels and constricting, pointed toe-boxes are the most common victims. I have yet to meet such a woman who can go five years without acquiring a deformed fifth toe.

The third-most-common cause of hammer toe is *pes cavus,* or claw foot. This is medicalese for a foot so excessively arched that it is almost S-curved. The excessive arch causes tightened tendons in the entire foot and results in contraction of all five toes. A claw foot is usually congenital, but it can be caused on rare occasions by a neuromuscular disease or by a trauma that affects the neuromuscular system of the foot. People who suffer from this condition have a difficult time finding shoes that are both comfortable and fashionable.

The fourth, and rarest, cause of hammer toe is neurological dysfunction in the foot, which can lead to contracture of the muscles and an abnormally high arch. Fortunately, I have seen few such cases in my years of podiatric practice. I say "fortunately" because these problems are generally quite difficult to treat. They are manifestations of systemic disorders that are often difficult to trace without expensive, uncomfortable, time-consuming testing. When these rare cases do occur, they are best referred to a neurologist for a complete evaluation.

How Hammer Toes Cause Corns

Now that you know the causes of hammer toe, we can once again turn our attention to corns. Just keep in mind the shape of the toe once it has been affected by tightening of the muscles and tendons: bent upward at the first joint (see Figure 5.1).

Once a hammer toe has formed, wearing a normal shoe will cause constant irritation to the elevated part of the toe. In order to prevent a serious inflammation from developing because of the irritation, a thickened layer of skin—a corn—will form on top of the toe.

If the corn were left alone, it would serve its protective purpose in peace and quiet. Unfortunately, however, the toe now has a large protuberance on top of a joint that is already bent upwards. This situation makes wearing shoes even more of a problem, because the corn itself is being irritated, and this irritation touches the nerve endings under the skin. The resulting pain will eventually force the sufferer of a hammer toe to seek medical attention.

The problem is not always confined to the affected toe. In order to alleviate pain from a corn without abandoning ill-fitting shoes, people will compensate by altering their gait to avoid pressure on the offending toe. After walking abnormally like this for a period of time, they will probably develop other biomechanical dysfunctions that could lead to problems in the lower limbs and even in the lower back.

The Case of the Invisible Roots

The fact that corns can create indirect problems elsewhere in the body reminds me of one of my favorite cases—and of the many myths concerning the causes and cures of corns.

I once had a patient who was suffering from knee pain that she believed was caused by a corn on her second toe. When I asked how she arrived at that diagnosis, she replied immediately that the roots of her corn had wrapped themselves around the insides of her foot, all the way up her leg to her knee, thus providing the "root" cause of her knee pain.

I did my best to keep a straight face and tried diplomatically to refute her theory. But she responded by insisting that I remove the corn so that I could see for myself. To calm her, I did remove the corn tissue, and then tried to show her that it had no roots. However, she was far from convinced.

"The reason you can't see the roots," she said, after some thought, "is that they are invisible. But I know you removed them as well. I can feel it."

The woman had no idea that I had trimmed her corn only superficially. But, since she appeared to be relieved and satisfied, I did not attempt to reason with her further.

A few weeks later this same lady was back in my office, this time for removal of an ingrown toenail. I inquired as to the health of her knee and was surprised and pleased to learn that within one week of the removal of her corn, her knee pain had disappeared.

This patient may have had the wrong self-diagnosis—corns definitely do not have roots—but she was quite accurate in assuming that her corn contributed greatly to her knee pain. As I mentioned above, when a corn or any other foot disorder causes pain in the foot, the sufferer logically enough begins to walk differently to remove pressure from the sore area. The altered gait produces either excessive pronation or excessive supination, either of which can result in knee pain. When the cause of the pain is removed, the reason for the abnormal gait is eliminated and the once-afflicted person returns to a normal biomechanical state of walking or running. Shortly thereafter, the knee pain will disappear. If it does not, the problem is probably not directly related to the foot.

My misinformed patient had no desire to learn the truth about her knee pain; she was adamant in sticking to her theory that invisible corn-roots were the cause of her discomfort. And if she keeps her corn properly trimmed, her knee pain may never return.

Treating Hammer Toes and Corns on Top of the Foot

So how can we remove a corn and thereby relieve the often excruciating pain that accompanies it? Well, as you might have guessed, there are both conservative and invasive methods, and treatment is often determined by the general physical condition and age of the patient, the degree of dysfunction and discomfort, and the patient's lifestyle.

Aside from the idea of excising the mythical roots of a corn, there are a few other old wives' tales about how to get rid of stubborn corns. In rare cases, some of the remedies even work, for reasons I will probably never understand. But I guarantee you that none of them will work permanently.

Beware of Home Remedies

Like some callus sufferers, there are people who frequently purchase small bottles of corn remover at their local pharmacies. The problem with this supposed wonder cure is that it is made of a powerful acid that can burn away not only corns and calluses, but surrounding normal skin as well. Moreover, people often hold to the principle that four drops are twice as effective as two, but all they are doing is doubling their trouble. Over the years I have treated a multitude of patients who had first-degree burns acquired by applying an extra-strength dose of corn remover. Unfortunately, the majority of these patients are older people, who seem to be more ready to accept home remedies and less enthusiastic about seeking medical attention for their foot problems—until they are in dire straits.

Too many elderly people, and even some of their juniors, also believe that if they cannot see the medication, it will not harm them. So they buy acid-treated pads to cover their corns or the calluses on the bottom of their feet. In about ten days they remove the pad, along with the corn, plus healthy skin that has been burned off. They are left with a nastily infected skin ulcer that will require medical treatment, and can be quite dangerous for those suffering from diabetes and/or circulatory disorders.

The production and sale of corn pads and corn removers has become a billion-dollar business over the years, and they can provide temporary relief for a minor case of corns. But, to repeat ad nauseam, the corns will return as long as the underlying cause remains. And as the corn recurs, the patient will increasingly use the acid treatments, often to the point where the skin has been burned right through to the underlying tissue. The burned skin and tissue are then exposed to bacterial infection as the wound ulcerates. The fault lies not with

the corn pad or the acid corn remover, but with the user who is trying to eliminate the "root" problem.

I strongly urge people who wish to use medicated corn pads and corn-removal liquids to apply them with discretion. If you are a diabetic or suffer from any kind of circulatory problem in your lower limbs, avoid them like the plague!

Another home remedy that can have severe consequences is using a knife or a razor blade to perform "bathroom surgery" to cut out a corn. Over the years I have seen quite a few cases where people took a shower or a bath, then used a sharp instrument to cut out a corn—along with a good deal of normal tissue. I can recall at least seven patients I had to stitch up after their clumsy attempts at bathroom surgery. A few of them actually reached the tendon before they discovered how deeply they had cut.

Safe, Conservative Approaches

A classic conservative approach to the treatment of corns, particularly those caused by hammer toes, is to wear specially designed deep shoes that provide far more space for the forefoot than do regularly cut shoes. The extra room in the toe-box prevents the hammer toe from rubbing against the top of the shoe. It is that friction, you will recall, that causes formation of the corn. The major problem with this approach is cosmetic, as the shoes tend to be particularly unattractive. Yet I strongly recommend them for people who have severe hammer toes but are poor candidates for surgical correction of their problem. I am referring mainly to those with poor circulation in their legs and feet, and particularly people who are elderly and generally not in the best of health. Let me remind those of you who are reluctant to give up high-fashion footwear that, despite the discomfort, it is far easier from a medical standpoint to change the shape of the shoe than it is to change the shape of the foot to fit a more aesthetically pleasing shoe.

Another conservative approach to alleviating the discomfort of a corn is the use of moisturizing creams and pumice stones, although they are generally beneficial only when soft corns are involved. Moisturizing creams may indeed be better for the feet than for the face. Application in the morning and evening of any cream sold over the cosmetic counter will work to keep corns soft and less painful.

Using a pumice stone after showering or bathing will reduce the thickness of dead skin. This makes more room for the toes inside the shoe and reduces pressure on the corn—and thus on the irritation. Again, keep in mind that creams and pumice stones will only alleviate the condition; the cause of the corn will still remain.

One conservative treatment is of some benefit to people who are poor surgical risks and who ought to avoid medicated corn pads and corn-removal liquids at all costs. It involves the use of a *buttress pad*. This pad elevates the offending toe by slipping around it. The pad cushions the toe from above and below and also serves to straighten out mild hammer-toe conditions. The buttress pad, along with a monthly trimming of the corn by an expert, will alleviate much of the discomfort. It ought to be the prime form of treatment for diabetics and for the elderly, who are generally most at risk from surgical intervention and the use of acid-based pads. Many new pads on the marketplace use gels that cushion the protuberance and can give temporary relief.

Surgical Remedies for Hammer Toes and Corns

For some people the surgical approach is the best answer. In this category are people who are unable or unwilling to put up with a certain amount of discomfort and who demand immediate relief without having to change the style of shoes they wear.

There are many sophisticated surgical techniques for eliminating hammer toes and the corns that develop on top of them. The least involved is called the *soft-tissue release*, or *plantar set*, procedure. The incision causes a minimal amount of trauma to the area, although diabetics and others with circulatory problems may still be poor candidates for the operation. This technique can be used successfully only when the two tendons above and below the bone are tight in the area of the hammer toe, but the bones themselves are normal. This is most often the case in the early stages of development of a hammer toe.

The soft-tissue release is a minimal-incision (MIS) procedure done under a local anesthetic, usually in a doctor's office. A tiny instrument is used to cut the offending tendon(s) via the underside of the deformed toe. Once the tendons have been cut, the toe automatically straightens out, eliminating the hammer shape. Although they have been severed, the ends of the cut tendons will eventually lengthen and reattach to each other without further medical intervention. It takes from six to twelve months for this to happen. Usually the incision is so small that stitches are not required, and postoperative discomfort is minimal. The success rate for this procedure is quite high.

The soft-tissue-release operation normally works quite well as long as bone in the area has not been deformed. The technique is ill-advised if there is a bone deformity, since the toe will still not straighten out. If a bone is involved, the surgeon must proceed to Plan B.

Plan B involves a procedure called *arthroplasty,* a word that means "surgically remodeling a joint." Arthroplasty can be either closed or open, depending on the condition of the toe joint and/or the technique preferred by the surgeon.

Communication between doctor and patient is important before surgery. The patient must understand that if part of the proximal phalanx has to be removed, the toe from which the offending corn was taken will be slightly shorter. Or, in the case of a soft-tissue-release procedure, the newly shaped toe will appear to be slightly longer because the offending tendon(s) will have been cut, thereby releasing the pulling effect on the toe joint. Many patients, unaware that their surgically treated toe might end up with a new shape, become needlessly upset after the operation because they had expected it to make the toe perfectly symmetrical with the others. Such is not the case. The surgeon's goal was to remove the cause of the irritation and return the foot to a condition where weight bearing is properly distributed throughout the foot.

After hammer-toe and corn-removal surgery, it is necessary to wear proper shoes so that the toes are not scrunched together and/or irritated again by shoes that are too shallow for the foot.

Soft-Core Corn

So far in this chapter I have concentrated primarily on the causes and treatment of corns that sit on top of the toes. These are hard layers of dead, thickened skin that form to protect the irritated part of a hammer toe from becoming even more inflamed. However, corns also form on the sides of the toes. Because they are kept moist by perspiration between the toes, they are called soft or wet corns. However,

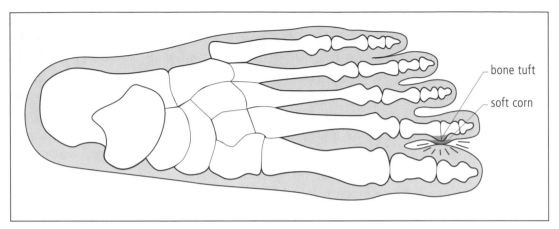

Figure 5.2. Formation of a soft corn

despite their name, they are hard—much harder than normal skin—and they can be far more painful than corns on top of the toes because of their proximity to nerves that run along the insides of the toes. The friction caused by a toe rubbing against a corn can irritate these nerves fiercely. And if one is unlucky enough to have corns on adjacent sides of two toes, the "kissing" corns constantly rubbing against each other can multiply the discomfort exponentially.

Whatever these soft corns are called, there is no mistaking the fact that they can produce exquisite pain. They are usually caused by a bony growth that causes the toe to jut out, and this results in friction with the adjacent toe (see Figure 5.2). The condition is exacerbated by wearing shoes that are too tight in the front. Once the soft corn has fully flowered, even properly fitting shoes will cause irritation, because the inflamed area is so sore that even a minor amount of friction will cause the nerves of the toe to be irritated.

Although it is obvious that scrunched toes are squeezed together by tight shoes, it is not quite so clear why the bony deformity that causes the corn to develop occurs in the first place. It is generally thought to be caused by a biomechanical fault combined with too tight a shoe, which forces the offending toe to curl sideways. Instead of being transformed into a hammer toe, the offending toe lies up against an adjacent toe in an awkward position. As in the development of a bunion, the bone is forced to jut out. It then becomes irritated, and subsequently a corn forms to protect it.

Treatment of Soft Corns

If the soft corn is newly developed and quite mild, treatment is quite simple. The corn is trimmed and a donut pad is applied to protect the area. At the same time the patient is strongly urged to switch to more comfortable shoes to avoid further problems. Unfortunately, not all my patients comply with that suggestion.

For my more recalcitrant patients, I am eventually obliged to take more vigorous action to treat their soft corns. I also see new patients whose soft-corn problems are beyond the stage of nonsurgical treatment. Rest assured, though, surgery for these types of corns is minor, performed using an MIS technique that does not involve much time or discomfort on the part of the patient.

The procedure is called *exostectomy,* and it involves shaving down the protruding bone with a burr that is introduced through a small stab incision in the toe. The surgery is done in a doctor's office under a local anesthetic, and requires only a stitch or two to close the wound made by the incision. After the operation the patient can walk out of the office fairly easily and return to normal activity, as long as they are not required to spend a lot of time on the feet for the rest of the day. This procedure is performed by almost all foot surgeons, even those who normally use only open techniques, because it is quite a simple operation.

Between a Nail and a Hard Place

One other type of corn that can be a real pain is the *subungual heloma* (medicalese for "corn under the nail"). It is caused by a small tuft of bone that forms at the end of the toe bone under the nail. The bone tuft develops either because of a trauma to the offending bone—particularly in the case of youngsters—or as a result of some hereditary quirk.

The common complaint is of pain in the nail area of the affected toe. The patient will say that it feels like an ingrown nail or as if something were growing under the nail. The reason for this is the direct pressure being brought to bear on the soft tissue between the tuft of bone and the nail. This pressure is being caused by the squeezing of the tissue in a cramped space, often by shoes that may be too tight. To help alleviate this sensitivity and to protect the bone tuft, a corn forms under the nail bed where the pressure is being felt. The corn makes the space between the bone tuft and the nail even more cramped, and the pain increases.

The condition can occasionally be relieved by a simple change of footwear. It is possible to avoid irritating the area by wearing shoes that fit properly in the toe-box. However, most of the time the problem has been allowed to develop over a long period of time because it was misdiagnosed as a fungal nail or something similar.

If a simple change of footwear fails to provide relief, there are two ways of treating a subungual heloma. If the condition appears to have been caused by an isolated traumatic incident, the solution is to remove the corn surgically. This can be done in a doctor's office under a local anesthetic, and the patient will be able to walk immediately after the corn has been removed.

The operation involves removing an overlying piece of nail, then excising the corn beneath it.

If the corn recurs repeatedly, the bone tuft itself should be removed. This procedure can also be done in a doctor's office under a local anesthetic. Discomfort to the patient is minimal, and he or she ought to be able to walk easily out of the office after the operation has been completed. The nail itself is left untouched. The success rate of this type of closed procedure is very high.

Baby Blues

The baby, or fifth, toe is particularly susceptible to corns, both hard and soft. Most of the time the corns, which may develop on the top or on either side of the toe, are created by shoe pressure. There is simply too little space in the toe-box to accommodate the baby toe, which is then twisted and contracts over a period of years until the top of the toe appears to be on the outside. This condition is called an *axially rotated toe*. An axially rotated baby toe is also being squeezed by the toe next to it. As a result, corns develop, and they can be excruciatingly painful—as many of my patients are all too eager to tell me.

If the more comfortably fitting shoes and/or corn pads do not sufficiently alleviate the discomfort, surgery is required. Once again, it can easily be performed in a doctor's office under a local anesthetic. Basically, the axially rotated baby toe has to be derotated, that is, moved back into its normal shape. The patient suffers little discomfort following the operation and is able to walk immediately. Assuming that the surgery is properly performed and the patient follows the postoperation care rules, recovery will take no more than a few weeks.

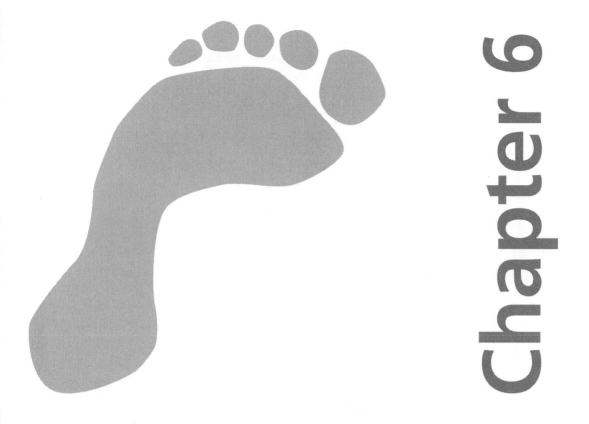

Calluses
and Warts

Chapter 6: Calluses and Warts

The soles of the feet support the full weight of the body, which creates constant pressure when you are standing. In addition, numerous sensory nerves are located close to the surface of the soles. It is not surprising, then, that irritation to the bottom of the foot can result in excruciating pain.

When Abe Lincoln complained publicly that his feet hurt, he may well have been referring to the soles of his feet, because that is where we most generally feel the strain of a hard day, particularly if we have been "running around" or standing for hours on end in less than perfectly comfortable footwear. Tired feet may cause you some dismay, but you can always soak them in a soothing tub to relieve the ache. By the end of this chapter you will be able to distinguish between feet that are merely tired and those that require professional attention.

The Callus Versus the Wart

Before proceeding to descriptions and treatments of calluses and warts, I will briefly explain the difference between the two. Warts are generally quite distinct in appearance from calluses. The primary difference is the presence of blackish pin dots (papillae) on warts that are not found on calluses. Also, certain calluses have a whitish center core, or nucleus.

The causes of the two disorders are as different as night and day. A wart develops after the foot has been invaded by a virus. A callus develops, like a corn, in response to pressure on a specific area of the sole of the foot. The pressure is caused by poor weight distribution due to a biomechanical fault. As you can well imagine, treatments for the two disorders are as different as their causes; the only thing a callus and a wart have in common is their location on the bottom of the foot.

The Callus Truth

In medical folklore, calluses are often lumped together and confused with corns. Like corns, they are nothing more than a buildup of thick skin to protect a part of the body that is being subjected to undue stress—in this case, the ball of the foot, which is located under the heads of the metatarsal bones. People get calluses on their hands from manual labor. However, because they do not normally walk on their hands, these calluses do not hurt unless some other force, such as squeezing a tool or a golf club, stresses them. But when the bottom of the foot is subjected to the pressure of body weight while a person is standing or in stride, the area where the callus has formed will hurt, because the ultrasensitive sensory nerve endings that are so close to the surface layers of the skin become irritated.

It is imperative to understand that a callus is a symptom of a disorder, not the direct cause of your discomfort. As I have mentioned, the ubiquitous biomechanical fault is usually the problem; it can cause calluses on the bottom of the foot, particularly in the area shown in Figure 6.1. So, while you may want to have your callus permanently and immediately removed by some magic remedy, it is just not going to happen unless the underlying cause is also eliminated.

I won't even try to count the number of times patients have asked me to "get out all the roots" when I am removing their calluses. As with corns, there are no roots to cut out, and the calluses will reappear as long as excessive pressure—caused by poor biomechanical function—is being applied to that particular area of the bottom of the foot.

When it comes to the formation of calluses, the number-one enemy is abnormal pronation. As the foot rolls across the metatarsal heads, the weight of the body is distributed unequally on the separate heads, one at a time, rather than equally in conjunction with each other in a normal rolling motion. As you walk or run, at least one of the metatarsal heads, usually either the second or the fifth, receives the brunt of your weight with each step you take. This added stress on the burdened metatarsal head causes inflammation of the area, and a callus forms to protect the sore spot. Eventually the callus develops to a point where it becomes a problem; the buildup of thick, dead skin so close to the nerve endings on the underside of the foot begins to cause extreme pain.

Another one of the classic biomechanical causes of a callus is the plantar-flexed metatarsal head. As you will recall,

in this situation one of the metatarsal heads is lower than the other four heads. What happens is that the lower-sitting head winds up absorbing as much as 80 percent of the weight normally distributed in proper proportion across all the metatarsal heads. As a result, thickened skin—a severe *nucleated* callus—may develop to protect the area. This type of callus has a

Figure 6.1. Dropped metatarsal head and formation of a callus

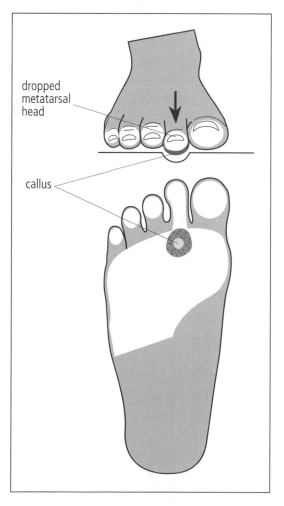

small white center core that represents the pinpoint-sized area of the metatarsal head where most of the excess weight is being absorbed (see Figure 6.1).

The position of the offending metatarsal head vis-à-vis the rest of the heads is crucial in determining the amount of buildup of callus tissue. The lower the abnormal position of the metatarsal head, the greater the development of callus tissue. If you have calluses all along the sole of your foot, it is obviously not because all the metatarsal heads are too low relative to each other. I suspect that your troubles have a different origin, more likely a different pronation abnormality combined with a compensatory forefoot deformity. Whatever the cause of the callus growth, however, the primary mode of treatment is correction of the biomechanical fault causing the problem.

The metatarsal head most likely to be affected is the second (corresponding to your pointing finger), followed by the fifth, then the third. Thanks to modern computer technology, weight distribution on the foot when a person is in stride can be precisely measured to determine the exact biomechanical problem—for example, the percentage of weight borne by each metatarsal head. With this information, the foot specialist can set out to normalize weight distribution on the foot during the gait cycle and eliminate both the cause and effect of the biomechanical fault. Of course, you already know the best early response to biomechanical problems that cause foot

troubles: wearing orthotics in the shoes. However, other treatments, depending on the severity of the condition, can be effective. I will examine all the forms of callus treatments shortly, but first I want to describe briefly remedies that ought to be avoided.

What Not to Do

Do not cut out calluses by yourself! You will suffer the same discomforts that you would with a self-excised corn. The symptoms will be relieved for a short time only, and bathroom surgery can lead to an unexpected visit to your local hospital for emergency treatment. If any lay (or professional) foot specialist suggests merely removing the thickened skin without treating the underlying cause of the callus, I suggest that you seek a second opinion.

Be wary of any exotic treatments that may be presented as options. I have seen patients who have undergone radiation treatment, surgery to remove the callus and its roots, plastic surgery to ostensibly make the area aesthetically pleasing, and even partial amputation to relieve the pain—and part of the foot. These radical options were presented to the patients without considering correction of the weight-distribution problem that probably caused the callus in the first place.

A callus is more than likely to respond best to conservative, noninvasive treatment. If you are presented with a radical approach to the removal of your callus before a conservative step has been taken, get a second opinion from another doctor, preferably one who specializes in feet.

The Right Step

Now that you know what not to do when you have a bothersome callus, you are ready for the next step—the right step. Once again our old friend the orthotic comes to the rescue. It works to eliminate the weight-distribution problem on the metatarsal heads, whether the condition is caused by a plantar-flexed metatarsal head, another biomechanical dysfunction, or a combination of disorders. If it is properly fitted, not only does the orthotic correct the weight-distribution discrepancy, it also serves to raise a low metatarsal head. Once the biomechanical fault has been eliminated, an ordinary callus will disappear slowly by itself, over a period of six to twelve months.

A nucleated callus, however, requires treatment on a regular basis every few weeks, even after the biomechanical cause has been eliminated by using an orthotic. This is because old customs are often hard to break, and the foot has been tricked by habit to form callus tissue. It may continue to do so even though the irritation no longer exists. The remains of the nucleated callus should be trimmed with a sharp knife by an expert. Once again, I cannot stress too strongly how dangerous it is for you to do this at home. The risk of cutting too deeply is real; the consequences are in-

fection and other damage to healthy tissue, and the possible formation of scar tissue.

If a severely plantar-flexed metatarsal head is causing a serious callus and if your quality of life is being adversely affected by the discomfort, surgery may be required to correct the malformation of the bone. The problem cannot be eliminated solely by wearing orthotics. As with much foot surgery, correction of a plantar-flexed metatarsal head can be done using either an open or closed (MIS) osteotomy procedure. Both can be performed in a doctor's office under local anesthetic. In either case, the risk of infection is minimal and the patient can walk immediately after the operation. However, the MIS technique appears to cause less discomfort, since the incision is smaller and there is less overall trauma to the area.

The success rate for plantar-flexed metatarsal-head surgery is about 80 percent. In the 20 percent of operations that fail, the problem is usually that the bone is raised too high relative to the adjacent metatarsal bones. You can guess what happens in that situation. One or two metatarsal heads, next to the one that was operated on, wind up too low relative to the others on the foot. On the bottom of the foot, under these newly affected metatarsal heads, you will soon discover that new calluses develop to protect the area from the stress of a too heavy weight load. You may have traded in one callus for another in a different area.

Whether the surgery is open or closed, how long does it take the foot to heal after a successful osteotomy? Providing that you take it easy—in other words, avoid running marathons or engaging in other strenuous physical activities until the area has healed—you should heal completely within six to twelve weeks. Assuming that the operation was a success, the callus should disappear in three to six months.

Sometimes a biomechanical fault can cause nucleated calluses under more than two metatarsal heads at one time. When this happens, surgical intervention (an osteotomy) will probably be required. While an orthotic may work well if only one or two bones are involved, it is much more difficult if more than two metatarsals are affected, because it is then much harder to equalize weight distribution. Too many abnormal metatarsal heads require equalizing. If orthotics fail to provide relief, the abnormal metatarsal heads that require equalizing may have to be surgically corrected to restore weight-distribution balance to the foot.

You may think by now that calluses occur under only the front part, or ball, of the foot. They are indeed most often found there, but they also occur, though less frequently, on the heel of the foot. So, before we tackle warts, we ought to take time to discuss callused heels.

The Callused Heel

The callused heel is the foot doctor's nemesis, because it is not easy to treat successfully. The calluses actually form around the edges of the heel, and rarely on the bottom. If you do discover something unusual on the bottom of your heel, it is most likely a wart, not a callus.

Unlike calluses on the soles of your feet under the metatarsal heads, calluses on the edges of the heel are not caused by a weight-distribution problem. They result from the combined effects of dry skin and constant irritation caused by an ill-fitting shoe. Orthotic devices to treat heel calluses will be useless, since the problem is not biomechanical. In fact, older types of orthotics may increase the irritation around the heel callus, thereby aggravating the problem. Mere trimming of the callus will provide relief for only a few weeks.

In more obstreperous cases, heel calluses can become so dry and hard that they crack. This results in a *lesion* (fissure) of the skin, and the area may bleed and become infected. If the fissuring is mild, apply a good commercial moisturizing cream to the affected area and then cover it with a wrapping of plastic film, such as Saran Wrap, to hold in the body's moisture. Leave the cream on all night, shower in the morning, and then use a pumice stone to smooth the callused area. With luck, you will experience relief in a few weeks.

If the condition is more severe, you will probably have to visit a foot specialist in order to prevent total breakdown and cracking of the skin, as well as the possible development of an infection at the site. Once the callused area has begun to improve—with the help of antibiotic cream, soaking, and use of a pumice stone—the doctor will more than likely tell you to revert to a daily application of moisturizing cream at home. If the problem is particularly difficult and serious infection develops, it may be necessary to take oral antibiotics.

In general, callused heels will not be miraculously cured overnight. Constant care and patience are the two ingredients most required to treat the condition. Anyone who has suffered through a lifetime of dry skin will understand the difficulty. Medical researchers are still searching for a panacea for many dermatological disorders, and dry skin anywhere on the body is no exception. As far as heel calluses are concerned, however, there is one thing anyone can do to improve the situation: Wear more comfortable shoes that do not irritate the sides of the heels.

Warts

Two different types of warts are found on the bottom of the foot and, less commonly, elsewhere on the foot. Both of them are caused by the *papilloma* virus. The most common wart is the *verruca vulgaris*—a combination of Latin and medicalese that means "common wart." The verruca vulgaris accounts for about 95 percent of all warts on the bottom of the foot. It occurs singly most of the time, although occasionally in clusters of five or six.

The other type of wart is called *mosaic verruca* because of its appearance. It usually occurs in clusters of fifty to sixty small growths in one concentrated area. Although it has not been scientifically proven, I suspect that mosaic verruca is caused by an offshoot of verruca vulgaris. The mosaic wart is far more difficult to treat than the common wart because the virus is much more widespread in the area and is not easily destroyed completely.

A Viral Attack

Contrary to popular fairy tales, warts are not caused by encounters with toads, a witch's curse, or abnormal behavior. The papilloma virus is solely to blame. This little devil, like all its cousins in the virus mafia, flourishes in all sorts of environments and can be picked up and transmitted by humans when the proper conditions exist. When the virus invades the bottom of the foot, a *plantar wart* will develop. It is called a plantar wart because it grows on the bottom, or plantar, part of the foot, not because it grows like a plant or is "well planted," with roots under the skin.

I believe that there must be a readily available blood supply to the area to allow a wart to grab hold and begin growing. So, while the papilloma virus may indeed be contagious, it only spreads when the proper conditions exist for it to find a new home. For a plantar wart to develop, the virus must enter the bottom of the foot through an abrasion or puncture wound, and there must be a good supply of blood to the site. Two other factors contribute to successful invasion of the virus. First, it requires both warmth and nourishment to flourish, and the bottom of the foot usually meets that requirement. Second, the virus has to outfox the body's natural immune system. Most experts—and most sufferers from plantar warts—will agree that the warts are very difficult to treat; viruses in general have been able to outsmart the natural defenses of many people and the research of medical scientists. Mankind is still waiting for a cure or prevention for the common cold, which is caused by a host of viral infections. In the past fifteen years we have learned how difficult it is to prevent or cure many deadly viruses, such as HIV, SARS, and a host of other diseases, such as West Nile and Ebola.

Once the virus that causes a plantar wart establishes a foothold, it spreads and multiplies to form a painful growth. It hurts so much because it usually finds a weight-bearing part of the foot to nest in. The small black dots that form on the surface of the wart are nothing more than tiny blood vessels that nourish it. Many people who look at these discolorations automatically assume that they are the ends of the "roots" of the wart. This is pure nonsense; warts no more have roots than do corns and calluses.

The papilloma virus is also very clever when it comes to self-preservation. It outsmarts the efforts of the body's natural de-fenses by forming a capsule around the developing wart. This encapsulation prevents the body's immune system from attacking and killing off the virus. The virus is quite content to remain in the superficial layers of the skin, so the wart does not penetrate very far below the surface of its host. However, the virus is so clever that it can somehow hide itself under the skin, even when the wart itself has been totally removed. This is why a wart can return in the very same spot where it originally developed.

Wart Removal

The best way to deal with plantar warts is to try to prevent them from developing in the first place. Since the virus will enter the skin through a wound of some kind, the logical solution is to prevent any lesions in the skin. Of course, that is not always possible.

Because of some of the reasons I have mentioned, once the virus has penetrated the skin on the bottom of the foot, it will be difficult to dislodge. Some viruses, including the papilloma variety, are like unwanted house guests who hang around underfoot until the host finally gathers the resources to strike back and force the unwelcome visitors to leave. During their stay, the intruders can create a fair amount of discomfort and may eventually have to be physically removed through the use of harsh measures. And they may return, despite all efforts to keep them away.

Naturally, you do not want to burn down the house to get rid of your unwanted guests (unless you need the insurance money). Neither do you want to destroy healthy body tissue on the bottom of your foot to get rid of a plantar wart. Keep this in mind as we discuss the various treatments. It is also important to consider that warts in general have a lifespan of about two years—although I have known some to hang around longer. Therefore, if you are not unduly distressed by the presence of a wart on your foot, or elsewhere for that matter, you could decide to let nature take its course.

Potatoes, Cod Liver Oil, and Other Snake-Oil Remedies

When it comes to the treatment of plantar warts, there are so many old wives' tales and new theories that they are almost impossible to catalog. It amazes me that so many of them occasionally seem to work, despite medical logic—which is downright embarrassing to the medical profession. My rule of thumb when dealing with plantar warts has become that if the cure is not potentially worse than the disease, by all means try it.

One of my patients had tried various home and medical remedies before he got rid of his plantar wart using hypnosis ther-

apy. It is apparently true that warts are susceptible to the power of suggestion. If that hypothesis is correct, it seems logical that hypnotic suggestion would work. It may also explain why putting potatoes or spitting saliva on a wart can make it go away. If you believe strongly in these cures, they could well be successful. But my studies and experiences have shown that the psychosomatic approach seems to work better when combined with more conventional treatment methods.

A few years ago I was on a radio talk show. In response to a question from a listener, I mentioned a supposed cod-liver-oil cure for plantar warts. Within a few weeks I received numerous testimonials in the mail attesting to the fact that the cod-liver-oil treatment really works.

I am sure there are many other harmless treatments, old and new, for getting rid of plantar and other warts. If I wanted to devote an entire chapter—even a book—to such remedies, I am certain that I would have no trouble doing so. But now I will examine the conventional ways of permanently removing plantar warts.

Acids

Numerous acid products for the treatment of warts are sold over drugstore counters, and doctors use more potent acids than those that are readily available to the public. These solutions are generally considered to be effective in only about 60 percent of cases. The percentage may actually be slightly higher, since doctors usually see only people who have failed to gain relief from over-the-counter preparations.

A doctor uses a 60 percent salicylic-acid solution that is available either in a cream or on medicated pads. This acid is applied twice daily. After showering, you smooth the affected area with a pumice stone to remove layers of the wart. Eventually you will reach the bottom of the wart. By removing all the layers, you may be lucky enough to kill the papilloma virus completely, and the wart will never return.

There are also acid-plaster dressings that can be applied weekly to a wart. Once a week the wart is peeled off, layer by layer, until there is no friendly environment left in which the virus can thrive. Unfortunately, this works only about 50 to 60 percent of the time. The papilloma virus is extremely adaptable, even in hostile environments.

One problem with using over-the-counter or prescription acid treatments is the temptation to abuse the remedy. If one drop is good, you may think two ought to be better and quicker, and ten ought to be fantastic. Of course, what happens with overapplication of an acid is a nasty acid burn. Also, lacking medical direction, you might be using an over-the-counter preparation for warts when the problem is actually a callus, which has

to be treated as a biomechanical dysfunction of the foot. Warts treated as calluses, on the other hand, rarely respond positively unless a callus has developed around the wart to protect the area from its painful pressure. In that case, the treatment indicated is twofold: biomechanical correction for the callus, and topical medication for the wart.

Freeze!

Liquid nitrogen works a little like both a laser beam and an acid. Because its temperature is so low (−465°F), when it is applied to a wart it freezes (or burns, or vaporizes) the growth, which then blisters and can be peeled away in layers until only the bottom layer remains. A final application of liquid nitrogen then removes the last of the wart and, we hope, the rest of the papilloma virus. Sad to say, this treatment works in only about 60 percent of the cases in which it is tried.

Surgery

If all of the above methods for nonsurgical removal of a plantar wart have failed and if the patient is suffering from unacceptable discomfort and dysfunction, it may be necessary to resort to excision. I want to emphasize, however, that surgery is often no more effective than any of the noninvasive treatments, and it could leave the patient with even more discomfort than he or she began with. This is because scar tissue may form where the skin has been cut, and this scarring can be very painful, since the patient will be constantly walking and putting pressure on the area. Another problem with surgery is that it can cause problems in patients who suffer from circulatory and/or other systemic disorders. Their healing will be much slower, and the risk of postoperative infection far greater, than in normal, healthy patients. For these reasons, I try to avoid operating on the bottom of the foot, whatever the problem, unless I have absolutely no choice.

Laser surgery is making quantum leaps, and there is much room for using lasers to treat foot problems that might normally require more invasive procedures. In the past few years, lasers have been used more often as a surgical tool for removing plantar warts, and much research has been done on laser surgery since I wrote my first foot-care book in 1985. However, there is no evidence to date that such a procedure is any more effective for removing plantar warts than traditional surgery. Moreover, just as much scar tissue can form on the bottom of the foot postoperatively. So, I repeat, try to avoid any surgical procedures on the bottom of the foot if at all possible.

Wrapping Up the Wart

By now you may have decided what you are going to do if you are unlucky enough to develop a plantar wart—or a wart on any other part of the body, for that matter. You may have also realized that there is no surefire solution to the problem.

However, there is another option, as I mentioned earlier in the chapter. Most warts will go away by themselves—eventually. Some disappear in a matter of weeks without any treatment whatsoever, while others hang around for years. If you are a patient person who is not in great discomfort from your plantar wart, I suggest that you simply try to wait it out.

One step I strongly urge you *not* to take is to try to cut out the wart yourself. You could cause yourself a lot of grief by cutting too deeply, thereby creating an extensive amount of scar tissue and/or setting yourself up for a nasty infection. I cannot overemphasize the need to avoid bathroom surgery at all costs.

Finally, I want to remind you again, whatever steps you take, to make sure you know whether what you have on the bottom of your foot is a callus or a wart. If you fail to diagnose the disorder properly, your efforts to eliminate the problem by yourself will be unsuccessful.

Chapter 7

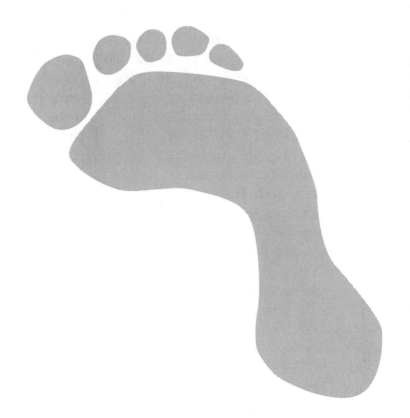

Disorders of
the Rearfoot

Somehow over the years, the poor down-trodden heel has acquired a bad reputation. In slang, a heel is a person who displays a shocking lack of decency or honor. In Greek mythology, another rear portion of the foot—the Achilles tendon—became synonymous with weakness. Nothing could be farther from the truth. The heel has tremendous shock-absorbing ability that protects the rest of the body from undue stress and is most important to one's gait. When you consider the constant pounding to which it is subjected—often on hard, uneven surfaces—over many, many years, it is amazing that the heel remains as healthy as it does.

However, if the rearfoot is injured in any way, it is often slower to heal (no pun intended) than other parts of the body because of the poor supply of blood to the area. For example, tendons will normally heal by themselves if ruptured (torn), but the Achilles tendon may have to be surgically repaired; too few fresh, healing nutrients reach its cells. With only a partial tear, however, the Achilles tendon can repair itself, and we are not so quick to take the patient to surgery. For the same reason, fractures of the bones in the back of the foot will also take longer to heal—and will be quite painful for longer. Fortunately, such fractures are rare, for reasons I will describe below.

As with other parts of the foot, there are quite a few myths floating around concerning the heel and what can go wrong with it and with nearby parts of the lower limbs. A lot of these old myths came under closer scrutiny when running and other exercises that place a lot of stress on the feet became more and more popular, and athletes began succumbing to rearfoot abnormalities. In my practice I now see many cases of heel and ankle-area injuries, and in a good number of these cases the patient has no concept of what the problem really is. And these patients are not alone; many medical professionals also have trouble diagnosing conditions affecting the rearfoot.

Incidentally, very little will be said in this chapter about the ankle. Although this joint is very sturdy and well designed, the wear and tear of athletic endeavors has resulted in a spate of ankle disorders among baby boomers. Years ago, almost all the ankle problems I saw were caused by trauma; for that reason, in my earlier books they were discussed primarily in the chapters on sports medicine. Now I am devoting part of Chapter 16, cowritten by Dr. Mark Myerson, a pioneer in foot and ankle surgery, to the overused and abused ankle.

There are numerous reasons for pain in the rearfoot, and in this chapter I intend to discuss the most common ones: plantar fasciitis, Achilles tendonitis, Haglund's deformity, and tarsal-tunnel syndrome.

The two major bones at the rear of the foot are the ankle bone (talus) and the heel bone (calcaneus). Together with other bones in the area they help form the *tarsus*—the rear part of the foot, including the ankle. When we have a sore heel, we most often blame it on a problem with the

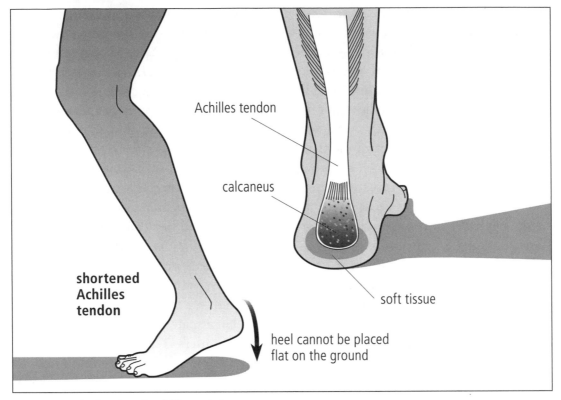

Achilles tendon

calcaneus

shortened Achilles tendon

soft tissue

heel cannot be placed flat on the ground

Figure 7.1. The heel and Achilles tendon

heel bone, but this is usually a misdiagnosis. The actual cause of the discomfort is not a bruise or a break in the bone, but inflammation of the adjoining soft tissue or pulling away of the periosteum (lining) of the bone.

Before we get to a discussion of inflammation of the soft tissues, we ought to examine the heel bone to understand why it is so difficult to injure it seriously. As you can see from Figure 7.1, the heel bone is a solid, block-like structure, well protected by the soft tissue that surrounds it and acts as a cushion. The bone can be broken or bruised, but only by a traumatic concus-

sive injury, such as a fall from higher than ten feet.

In all my years of practicing podiatry, I have seen a fractured heel bone only eight times. In the most severe case, a utility worker fell forty feet and landed on his heels on concrete pavement. I am sure he was much happier to have landed feet first rather than head first; a fractured heel bone may not heal any faster than a fractured skull, but there are generally far fewer side effects if the person survives the fall.

Another case was less serious, involving a rather comic—but potentially tragic—incident. One evening I was summoned to the emergency room of the hospital where

I worked as a resident to examine the foot of a middle-aged man. He had been forced to make a hasty retreat from the bedroom of his mistress when her husband returned from a trip much earlier than anticipated. The man had jumped out of the upstairs bedroom window and had been lucky enough to land feet first on the ground. He was so frightened that he ran for almost a mile before he realized that he had sustained a serious injury to the heel of one foot.

Breaching the Heel

If the heel bone rarely fractures or bruises, what causes heel pain? As I have already mentioned, in order to understand the cause of the discomfort, we have to look to the soft tissue in the area, particularly the plantar fasciae and the Achilles tendon.

As you can see from Figures 7.1 and 7.2, the heel bone is affected by the *Achilles tendon,* which is attached at the rear of the bone, and by the *plantar fasciae,* which are connected to the bottom front part of the bone. In a sense, the tendon and the fasciae compete with each other to influence the actions of the heel bone when a person is walking or running. When an abnormality occurs because one of these soft-tissue masses forces the other to overstress—for a variety of reasons, including poor biomechanics of the lower limbs—rearfoot pain occurs because of the resulting inflammation. The sufferer often believes that this pain comes from the heel bone.

Because the pulls of the plantar fasciae and the Achilles tendon are in ninety-degree opposing directions, it is not uncommon for both to become inflamed almost simultaneously, causing *Achilles tendonitis* (inflammation of the Achilles tendon) and *plantar fasciitis* (inflammation of the plantar fasciae). These two conditions are the main causes of rearfoot pain, so let us look at them in greater detail.

Plantar Fasciitis

Athletes, particularly runners, are well aware of the problem of plantar fasciitis, and I shall have much more to say about both athletes and athletic foot problems in Chapter 11. But, as with the general public, they do not really understand the disorder, and are saddled with numerous myths about how it is caused and how it ought to be treated. The plantar fasciae are attached to the heel bone and to the five metatarsal bones in the forefoot. The fasciae have two tasks to perform: The first is to support the longitudinal arch of the foot, and the second is to help prevent overpronation.

If the subtalar joint is pronating abnormally, the plantar fasciae, which in their normal condition are already tightly strung, become stretched even further and twist as they try to prevent the abnormal pronation. This extra stress can eventually cause the fasciae to pull the lining of the bone, the *periosteum,* away from the bone—a condition known as *periostitis* (inflammation of the lining of the bone).

Sufferers of this condition may experience excruciating pain when first getting out of bed in the morning. This is because the periosteum is like a Velcro attachment. The previous day, the periosteum has torn away from the heel. At night, while you are sleeping, it tries to reattach, but when you first step on it in the morning it starts to tear again. When this happens on a regular basis, you will become so uncomfortable that you will be forced to seek medical treatment. Depending on the expertise and discipline of the caregiver, you may be told that you are suffering from plantar fasciitis or—horror of horrors—heel spurs (more about heel spurs below). If you can imagine pulling a tuft of hair from your head, you will have a fair analogy to the discomfort of plantar fasciitis.

So, plantar fasciitis is usually caused by the fibers of the plantar fasciae tearing the periosteum away from the heel bone as they try to prevent the foot from over-pronating. However, abnormal pronation is not the sole cause of this condition. In the high-arched, semiflexible foot or the rigid foot, the plantar fasciae encounter added pressure to prevent the biomechanical problems associated with these conditions. Also, it appears that in older people the plantar fasciae tend to lose much of

Figure 7.2. The plantar fasciae

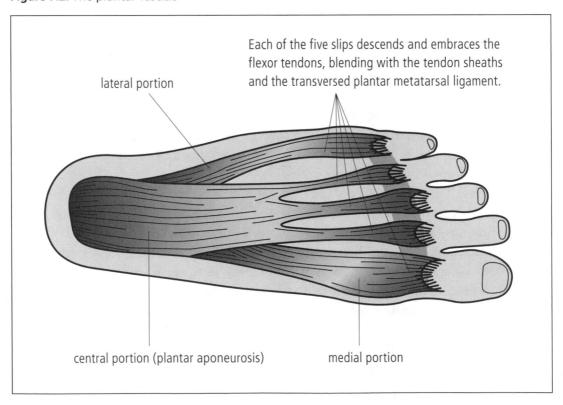

lateral portion

Each of the five slips descends and embraces the flexor tendons, blending with the tendon sheaths and the transversed plantar metatarsal ligament.

central portion (plantar aponeurosis)

medial portion

their elasticity, causing excessive strain to the area where the fasciae connect to the heel bone. As you might expect, as the area becomes inflamed, plantar fasciitis then occurs.

Plantar fasciitis can plague its victims for years. I had one patient who suffered from the disorder for twelve years prior to seeing me, during which time he had four operations to try to correct the problem. The surgery involved is quite controversial, and rarely warranted. This particular patient is now feeling much better thanks to advances in computer gait analysis and better orthotics, but he still has occasional recurrences of the disorder.

Spurring the Truth

Plantar fasciitis is often confused with heel spurs. I have lost count of the number of people who have told me that they suffer from heel spurs—because they were told so by another medical practitioner or by a friend with a similar problem. *People do not suffer from heel spurs, because heel spurs do not cause pain.* Spurs develop in response to a painful situation in an attempt to relieve the discomfort.

Heel spurs are not really spurs at all. When seen head on, they are ridges, although they may look like spurs in a two-dimensional X ray. Regardless of their appearance, their development can be explained by a simple theory of kinesiology: Bone conforms to the stress under which it has been placed.

When the plantar fasciae pull hard at the area where they are attached to the heel bone, the bone eventually begins to grow in the direction of the pull. This is nature's way of preventing the plantar fasciae from pulling the lining away from the bone. All things being equal, the inflammation around the stressed area will then heal. Unfortunately, however, this is not always the case.

In any event, it is the periostitis that causes the pain, not the bone, because bones have no pain nerve endings. Studies have shown that if both feet have heel spurs, the pain is much less noticeable when the ridge is longer.

Oh, How I Hate to Get Up in the Morning!

The classic characteristic of plantar fasciitis is pain in the area of inflammation when pressure is first put on the foot in the morning. Once a person with the disorder has been walking around for a few minutes, the pain subsides and normal daily routines can often be conducted without too much discomfort in the heel area. However, any lengthy time spent sitting or lying during the day will bring on the pain as soon as weight is again put on the foot. This is because the plantar fasciae are once more pulling the periosteum away from the bone.

Remember the Velcro analogy? One piece (the periosteum) has been reattached overnight to the fibers of the second piece (the plantar fasciae) in a normal healing process. Then in the morning, one step on the ground, and—rip! The two pieces are pulled apart again.

There is a second theory that also has merit. The plantar fasciae contract during the night when the feet are being totally rested, and are therefore very tight and sore when they are first subjected to weight bearing in the morning. As they stretch out naturally, the plantar fasciae become less stressed, reducing the pulling on the periosteum, and the pain subsides as the person continues to walk. This seems to be another plausible explanation of why the pain subsides after a few minutes of walking.

Becoming Well-Heeled: Part I

Successful treatment of plantar fasciitis is a double-barreled endeavor. On one hand, the inflammation must be dealt with; on the other, the cause of the disorder must be eliminated. In mild cases, elimination of the cause will eliminate the need for treatment of the inflammation itself. When the inflammation is more severe, it has to be attacked more vigorously.

For years it has been accepted practice to treat painful plantar fasciitis inflammations with injections of cortisone and a local anesthetic. The procedure often provides immediate relief that can last for six to twelve weeks, but the disorder will re-

turn because the cause of the problem will not have been eliminated. Because cortisone shots have side effects, as I have already mentioned, I have injected fewer than 5 percent of my patients. It is also fairly common today to prescribe oral anti-inflammatory drugs other than cortisone or similar steroids. However, all anti-inflammatory drugs have potential side effects that may outweigh the benefits in the long run. Moreover, no anti-inflammatory drug that I know of will by itself prevent abnormal pronation. However, if plantar fasciitis has been caused by a traumatic injury to the foot, such as a fall from a great height, an anti-inflammatory drug may clear up the condition on its own, since there is no underlying biomechanical fault in the foot.

In many cases where using an anti-inflammatory drug is not indicated, physiotherapy may help somewhat. Ultrasound is the treatment most often recommended. Icing the area may also help relieve the inflammation. However, physiotherapy on its own will not normally cure the condition. In those few cases where a biomechanical fault does not require using a special orthotic device, a simple, inexpensive arch support may make walking more bearable during the recovery stage.

In most cases of plantar fasciitis, however, the culprit is overpronation, and the treatment is a custom-made orthotic. Keep in mind, however, that the orthotic only prevents development of the condition; it does not relieve an inflammation that is severe enough to require painkilling treatment. Orthotics provide permanent long-term relief because they eliminate excessive torsioning of the plantar fasciae by preventing overpronation of the foot. When the foot no longer overpronates, there is no need for the plantar fasciae to overextend themselves to the point where they may tear the lining away from the heel bone. My experience has been that 90 percent of plantar fasciitis cases can be successfully treated by fitting proper orthotics. Even in severe, chronic cases when overpronation was excessive, an orthotic by itself did the trick, and the heel healed without needing drugs or physiotherapy.

It must be stressed, however, that orthotics do not provide *immediate* relief. It takes time for the plantar fasciae and the periosteum to heal and return to their normal condition. So you will have to be patient; eventually your heel will probably feel as good as new—if not better.

Athletes, and active people in general, are often hampered by soreness in the back part of their feet, and they resort to various types of heel cushions to protect themselves from their imaginary heel-spur disease. These foamy cushions make a regular appearance in my office, since most of my patients with plantar fasciitis wear them in their shoes constantly, in the mistaken belief that they will provide relief. Well, if they work, why are all these people in my waiting room?

Heel cushions do not work for plantar fasciitis because they do nothing to prevent overpronation. As a first step, I may suggest that my patients save their money to buy an inexpensive pair of properly constructed, perfectly fitting running shoes with a proper arch support and perhaps an anti-roll bar (not the kind found in racing cars) that acts to prevent overpronation. These shoes will not provide a 100-percent cure for plantar fasciitis, but in many instances they will help.

One of the stranger foam-padded cushions I have seen has its middle cut out in a donut shape, to protect the "painful" heel spur. The cushion is quite useless from this point of view, as it has absolutely no effect on the ridge of bone. But it does accidentally help the plantar fasciae by supporting them at the front and alleviating their overstretching. In fact, if you were to combine the donut-shaped pad with a decent arch support, you would wind up with a piecemeal treatment that might actually provide relief.

Of my rare plantar-fasciitis patients who required surgery, one of them had suffered from the disorder for twenty-three years. His condition was exacerbated by an occupational hazard: As a utility worker, he was constantly climbing up power poles, positioning his feet awkwardly to avoid losing his grip.

There are two separate surgical procedures for plantar fasciitis, both of which are done using MIS techniques. Whether the patient has heel spurs at the same time plays no role in either procedure. While I am not a proponent of surgery for plantar fasciitis, a new endoscopic surgery (done through a scope) removes the plantar fascia from its origin on the heel bone; in severe cases this treatment has been shown to be effective. However, this approach would be a last-resort treatment, used only after all else had failed.

The Achilles Heel

Achilles was a Greek hero of great acclaim as a warrior and healer. When he was a child, his mother, Thetis, took him by one heel and dipped him in the river Styx to make him physically invulnerable. But, unfortunately for the poor lad, the part his mother held remained dry, and therefore vulnerable. Eventually he was slain by the warrior Paris, who fired an arrow into Achilles' heel, the one weak spot on his body.

When medical professionals speak of Achilles, they refer not to the heel itself, but to the tendon that is a vital part of the rearfoot. We also tend to mutter under our breath when we run across a case of Achilles tendonitis, or inflammation of the Achilles tendon. The disorder is difficult to treat, particularly when we are dealing with an athlete who wants to rush back onto the field long before the inflammation has cleared up and who might be willing to risk regular recurrence of the problem in order to indulge in a favorite pastime.

However, it is not always the dedicated athlete whom we see with Achilles ten-

donitis. The most common victims, in fact, are women between the ages of twenty and forty-five. Some women begin wearing shoes with heels two to four inches high while they are still growing teenagers. They continue to wear high-heeled pumps as they enter the white-collar work force, because they do not want to look out of place in the office. As the years go by, these young women develop shortened Achilles tendons because the tendon no longer has to stretch to enable the foot to sit comfortably in a low-heeled shoe (see Figure 7.1).

But what happens when a woman who has been wearing high-heeled shoes almost exclusively throughout her mature years suddenly decides to go natural or become athletic, changing into low-heeled shoes for running, walking, or other activities? If her Achilles tendon has shortened substantially, she will not have the tendon length required to allow her foot to sit properly in the lower-heeled shoe. The tendon then tries to stretch to reach down the back of the foot, which is now positioned differently in relation to the lower leg. We saw what happens to the plantar fasciae when they are overstretched. The same happens to the Achilles tendon: It becomes overextended and twisted, pulling the periosteum away from the rear of the heel bone and causing periostitis—in this case, known as Achilles tendonitis.

Unless the problem is corrected, the condition will become chronic, particularly during the summer months, when the woman may be wearing sandals and casual shoes more often and regularly switching back and forth between high and low heels. As long as the woman continues to wear high-heeled shoes exclusively, she can avoid tendonitis. But of course, as you already know, high-heeled shoes can cause a host of other foot problems. (Incidentally, men who have worn boots with two-inch heels for their entire adult life and who then begin exercising in running shoes with one-inch heels may also develop an Achilles tendon problem.)

The second-most-common cause of Achilles tendonitis, one that affects both males and females, is congenital. Some babies are born with Achilles tendons that are too short, and they stay that way unless the situation is alleviated either by a program of stretching exercises or by surgery to lengthen the tendon. Tots who walk exclusively on their toes quite likely have Achilles tendons that are too short. In this case, tiptoeing has nothing to do with either stealth or speed.

The third-most-common cause of Achilles tendonitis is overstress of the tendon and the area surrounding it. This most often affects athletes and is a classic overuse syndrome. Overstressing of the tendon produces a periostitis inflammation that tends to become chronic because the athlete fails to rest or treat the traumatized area sufficiently. The condition is often exacerbated by a biomechanical fault, particularly abnormal pronation, that is ignored until the inflammation becomes severe. Occasionally the injury to the Achilles tendon is made worse by some traumatic episode, such as the sufferer taking a bad step and "turning" the ankle. Of course, such an accident can also strike the nonathlete, who may slip on a stair or a curb, landing one foot awkwardly on the step below and badly pulling the Achilles tendon.

As I mentioned above, Achilles tendonitis is an inflammation caused by overstretching and twisting of the Achilles tendon, which then pulls the lining of the bone away from either the back of the heel bone or at the place where it becomes the lower end of the two calf muscles—the *gastrocnemius* and the *soleus*. In some cases the fault is not that the Achilles tendon is overstressed or too short, but that a shortened calf muscle forces the tendon to overstretch to make up for the imbalance.

There are numerous ways of determining the cause of the tendonitis, and much of the diagnosis is based on the patient's medical history. Has the problem existed since childhood? Is there a history of the condition in adulthood? Has the problem begun since an athletic endeavor was undertaken? Has the patient recently switched from predominantly high-heeled shoes to low-heeled shoes? Has the patient suffered some sort of traumatic injury? Another important factor to be considered is abnormal pronation or abnormal supination. Are faulty biomechanics to blame for the disorder, either separately or in conjunction with another cause?

How can the ubiquitous biomechanical fault cause Achilles tendonitis? When the Achilles tendon fires (is activated), it pulls the foot into plantar flexion; that is, it lowers the front part of the foot toward the ground. When a person is running or otherwise engaged in athletic activities, the calf muscles act to decelerate the lower leg and foot; that is, when the heel is planted on the ground, the calf muscles prevent the lower leg from going forward too fast and causing an imbalance. This action of the calf muscles strains the Achilles tendon—but not abnormally, unless there is a problem. This problem could be either abnormal pronation or abnormal supination of the foot that tilts the heel bone to the inside or the outside. When this happens, the Achilles tendon will be pulled, perhaps beyond its comfortable limit, to compensate for the tilting heel bone. At the Sports Medicine Clinic at Toronto's Mount Sinai Hospital, I have seen this syndrome often, particularly in runners and tennis players, for reasons I shall discuss fully in later chapters.

Pain in the Achilles tendon will vary in location depending on where the inflammation and/or tearing is occurring. If the tendon is being overstressed where it joins with the two calf muscles, the discomfort will be felt in the lower leg; if the problem exists where the tendon attaches to the heel bone, the pain will be felt in that area. The worst possible thing that can happen to the Achilles tendon is a rupture, either complete or partial. When the tendon is torn in half, according to many victims, the sensation is one of being shot in the back of the leg; they also report hearing a loud "pop" when it happens. The pain is accompanied by a feeling of paralysis in the lower leg and foot, since the severed tendon is no longer able to provide essential locomotion for the lower limb. Many athletes have had their careers interrupted for a long time, or ended abruptly, by such an injury. When Al Gore was vice president of the United States, he was on crutches for quite a while after such a trauma.

Becoming Well-Heeled: Part II

As I mentioned earlier in this chapter, treatment of an Achilles tendon problem is not easy, primarily because poor blood supply to the area prevents essential nutrients from reaching the soft tissues in sufficient amounts to promote healing. So how do you get rid of the inflammation?

After the proper diagnosis and cause of the disorder has been established, the first course of action is therapy. A treatment method that has gained favor in the past few years is friction rubs, particularly for chronic conditions. Friction rubs work like some forms of massage, particularly shiatsu, and in fact inflame the sore area even more. The idea is to trick the body into attacking the inflammation with added vigor. Theoretically, if this happens, the inflammation will heal faster on its own, without the need for other forms of treatment. I believe that this is another positive example of making nature do the work that is often left to medication and direct intervention.

Once mechanical evaluation of the problem has been completed, orthotics have been prescribed when necessary, and therapy—whatever the form—has succeeded in calming the inflammation, stretching exercises can begin to lengthen both the Achilles tendon and the calf muscles, if that is necessary. However, it would be wise to warm up the muscles and the tendon first, for two reasons. Soft tissue that is cold can be damaged if stretched too far, and warm soft tissue can be stretched to its maximum, allowing for optimum results in the stretching program. Your therapist will show you how to do these exercises properly.

One method of treatment I avoid is using anti-inflammatory drugs, either injection of cortisone into the inflamed area or oral nonsteroidal pills. Cortisone injected into the area of the Achilles tendon may get rid of the inflammation, but it could also fray it badly, causing the tendon to rupture. And, because of the poor circulation to the area, I feel that oral anti-inflammatory drugs rarely benefit the patient, as the dosage level would have to be relatively high to get enough of the medicine to the limited blood supply in the area.

In extreme cases—usually when athletes afflicted by Achilles tendonitis refuse to rest—where the usual conservative treatments have not worked, it may be necessary to completely immobilize the tendon by placing the lower leg and foot in a cast. This prevents the patient from doing any more damage to the area and allows the Achilles tendon an opportunity to heal. The cast may have to be left on for six to twelve weeks, depending on the severity of the damage. A lengthy physiotherapy program will be required after the cast has been removed so that the tendon and the surrounding muscles can regain their normal strength and flexibility.

The only other time the area may have to be placed in a cast is if the Achilles tendon has been ruptured. If the tendon is severed it will have to be surgically sewn together, because poor blood circulation to the area will hinder natural healing. Once the surgery has been completed, the leg will be placed in a below-knee cast to prevent any motion of the tendon for about six to eight weeks while the area heals. As you can imagine, a lengthy physiotherapy program will follow.

Let us assume that the damage is not so severe and that the inflammation has been controlled by therapy and rest. What happens when the primary cause of the inflammation is determined to be biomechanical? Well, you have probably guessed that an orthotic device should be prescribed and put in the shoe as quickly as possible to prevent further inflammation. Orthotics are not total cures, because the tendon must still be stretched to normal length. However, these devices allow the tendon to pull at the proper angle relative to the heel bone and the calf muscles, because they correct the abnormal pronation or abnormal supination that has been causing the inflammation.

Since I began practicing podiatry and sports medicine, I have treated hundreds of cases of Achilles tendonitis with orthotics in conjunction with therapy. In these cases the patients had suffered the condition for at least one year without achieving relief from other treatments. My success rate has been over 85 percent.

The Cinderella Syndrome

We are all familiar with the story of Cinderella, the poor waif whose life changed dramatically when a piece of footwear transformed her miserable existence into one of love and luxury. What the fairy tale did not tell you is that whenever she wore her glass slipper, she endured a great deal of anguish, because it irritated the back of her foot terribly. She may well have been the first celebrity known to have suffered from "pump bump" (in medicalese, *Haglund's deformity*), a condition caused by irritation of the Achilles tendon area of the foot. The primary suspect is the pump—a shoe with two- to four-inch heels that is low-cut and has no straps or ties. While these shoes continue to be fashionable, they are hardly practical when foot comfort is involved.

The back of the offending shoe is usually slightly curved to cut directly into the back of the heel bone, which may already be under some stress from having an abnormally short Achilles tendon pulling on it. With plantar fasciitis, the front part of the heel develops a ridge, or spurs, to shorten the distance between it and the metatarsal heads. A similar *exostosis* (protuberance of bony or cartilage-like material) may form at the back of the heel to compensate for stress on a short Achilles tendon. This benign growth is called a pump bump, and an inflammation can develop because of the constant irritation of the area around the bump. This irritation is normally the result of pump-style shoes or, in a few cases, ski boots or skates. In any event, about 95 percent of the cases of pump bump I see are in women.

The inflammation caused by a pump bump can occasionally occur not only to the heel bone itself and/or to the Achilles tendon, but also to the bursa in the area. A *bursa* is a small sac of fibrous tissue that is filled with fluid. It acts to protect parts of the body that would otherwise be irritated by friction or by some other abnormal internal or external pressure, usually occurring between tendon, or other soft tissue, and bone (for example, in joints). However, the bursae can themselves become inflamed, and the result is *bursitis,* a condition that can produce sharp pain and tenderness in the afflicted area.

Two types of bursitis can occasionally affect the area around a pump bump: *retro-calcaneal* and *subcutaneous*. The former occurs between tendon and bone, and the latter between tendon and skin. These conditions are not easy to distinguish from Achilles tendonitis, and the senses and knowledge of an experienced foot specialist are often required to make the proper diagnosis. Bursitis in this part of the body can be treated by ice and ultrasound—and by wearing proper footwear, since the condition is exacerbated, if not directly caused, by shoe pressure that pushes tendon against bone or other soft tissue.

When the problem is with the pump bump itself, rather than the bursa, treatment is generally much the same: ice, ultrasound, and a change of footwear. Another possibility is a donut pad that can be applied directly to the sore area at the back of the foot or to the shoe, ski boot, or skate. This will alleviate pressure being applied directly to the inflammation. I know many athletes who wear these pads regularly to protect themselves from pump bump. An orthotic device may also be indicated if the condition involves an Achilles tendon that is too short, affecting the biomechanics of the lower leg and foot.

In very rare cases—about 2 percent of the time—surgery will be required to rid the patient of the inflammation. Usually the offending bump of bone is removed by filing it down. The procedure can be done under a local anesthetic in a doctor's office or surgery center, using either an open or an MIS technique. Recovery is normally quite rapid and uncomplicated.

In even rarer cases in which the Achilles tendon has actually attached to the heel bone where the pump bump developed, the tendon will have to be removed surgically from the bone and then reattached after the bump has been filed down. As you can imagine, this is a more complicated procedure, and to facilitate healing, the foot will have to be placed in a cast for six to twelve weeks. Before you begin to worry about this happening to you, be comforted by the fact that this type of surgery is required in less than 1 percent of all incidents of pump bump, and the condition is totally preventable.

The Dark at the Middle of the Tunnel

We come now to a nerve impingement condition called *tarsal tunnel syndrome,* a lesser-known cousin of the notorious carpal tunnel syndrome that is the bane of those who spend too much time working with computer keyboards. The tarsal tunnel runs down the back part of the lower leg into the foot; it is a small, bony passageway for the posterior tibial nerve and the lateral plantar nerve.

The tarsal tunnel runs under the *deltoid*

ligament. When something is amiss with the ligament and it impinges on the tarsal tunnel, or if the tunnel is otherwise constricted, the posterior tibial nerve is squeezed and entrapped. The agitated nerve then begins to send out confusing signals to the brain: numbness, a feeling of pins and needles, burning sensations on the bottom of the foot, and/or a stabbing pain in the ankle area. Because of these vague, diffused symptoms, tarsal tunnel syndrome is difficult to diagnose, particularly since the symptoms are often nonexistent when the deltoid ligament is at rest (that is, when the person is not exercising or walking). The resting ligament will not impinge on the nerve as it passes through the tarsal tunnel.

The primary cause of tarsal tunnel syndrome is our old enemy, the biomechanical fault. When a foot is severely overpronating, the deltoid ligament is forced to assume an abnormal position to compensate. The ligament then pushes down on the tarsal tunnel, indirectly impinging on the tibialis posterior nerve and causing tarsal tunnel syndrome.

The second major cause of the disorder is systemic—actually, a whole host of systemic disorders that may be serious or mild, temporary or permanent. When an ankle swells because of water retention, poor circulation, or even pregnancy (when poor circulation in the pelvic area can result in similar difficulties in the lower limbs), entrapment of the nerve can occur because the space allowed for the tarsal tunnel has been restricted. Only about 25 percent of the cases I see in my practice are systemically induced. (I suspect, though, that an obstetrician would see a much larger number of systemically induced cases.)

As I have already mentioned, diagnosing the syndrome is a real pain—for the doctor. When the patient is resting, there is a good chance the problem will not be evident at all, since the deltoid ligament causing the discomfort is relaxed and therefore not stressing the tarsal tunnel. I often ask my active patients who experience the discomfort only when running or engaged in other exercise to go out and run or exercise and then return to my office once the pain begins—if they can make it back. I advise them to take taxi fare with them in case they manage to produce excruciating pain while trying to induce the symptoms. When the patients return in agony to my office, I am then more able to seek the cause of the problem by conducting various nerve-entrapment tests that are themselves relatively painless.

If I find that the problem is tarsal tunnel syndrome, and if the problem is obviously systemic and accompanied by swollen ankles, I send the patient on to be seen by other specialists for further diagnosis and treatment. If, on the other hand, I establish that the cause is biomechanical, I can begin treating the patient.

As you would suspect, the proper

treatment for biomechanically induced tarsal tunnel syndrome is correction of the biomechanical fault. If the condition is relatively mild, using a simple arch support and/or switching to a well-constructed running shoe (for the patient who does not generally need formal footwear) should do the trick. If the disorder is more severe, the patient will require orthotics. Because of poor blood circulation to the area, anti-inflammatory drugs are of little use to control the discomfort. If the ankle itself has become swollen after being injured in some way, physiotherapy, such as application of ice or ultrasound, may help.

Chapter 8

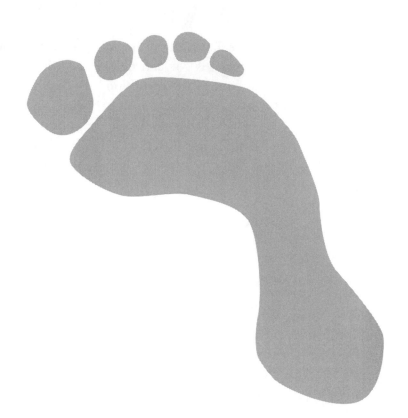

Children's Feet

Some of my most interesting patients are children, not only because they are likely to say and do the nuttiest things while in my office, but also because pediatric foot care, or *podopediatrics*, is often a challenging and very rewarding experience.

The first challenge of podopediatrics has to do with parental misconceptions about infant footwear and the development of a child's lower limbs. The second challenge is the inexperience of certain medical professionals in dealing with foot problems in infants, often because they lack sufficient training in podopediatrics to recognize a problem until it becomes blatantly obvious.

Before we look at specific foot problems affecting infants, it might be wise to differentiate between the normal and the abnormal foot during the growth of the limbs in the womb, and then from birth on. Thanks to the wonders of modern photographic techniques and computer technology, we have learned that the *limb buds*—the beginnings of the arms and legs—start to form about four weeks after conception. One week later, it should be possible to recognize the shape of the foot. By the twenty-sixth week, the embryonic foot should be fully developed. At birth, a normal infant who was delivered normally ought to have fully developed feet with all the soft-tissue formations, nerves, and circulatory system in place. All the bones are also present at birth, with the exception of the two end bones, the distal phalanges, of the baby toes. Naturally, the standard model includes five toes on each foot, complete with minuscule toenails. All the bones in the infant's foot will undergo changes in size, shape, and position as the foot prepares itself for weight bearing.

When a doctor is examining a newborn baby to determine whether or not the feet are normal, he or she must consider the lower limbs as complete units. It is vital to check the positioning of the foot vis-à-vis the overall shape of the leg and the positions of the hips and knees. Potential problems exist if the baby is decidedly bowlegged or knock-kneed. If these abnormalities are present, the foot of the child will be affected, particularly as it begins to walk and if the infant's legs are twisting internally or externally (internal or external torsion) the foot will either in-toe or out-toe to compensate.

After I examine the lower limbs as a whole, I turn my attention to the feet themselves. Because of the many intricate motions of the foot and ankle, it is not easy for a practitioner to tell the normal from the abnormal, and I am therefore very exacting in my manipulations. However, according to the most recent statistics, only one infant in a hundred who is a full-term baby and has had an uneventful delivery will suffer from an abnormal foot problem that requires immediate attention.

I always stress to new parents who have babies with normal feet that their children ought to be left alone to develop by themselves. I also tell these anxious parents what my pediatrics professor told me back in medical school many years ago: "If God, in his infinite wisdom, had meant babies to wear shoes, they would have been born with them." As far as pre-walkers are concerned, the only function of shoes is to keep a child's feet warm when necessary. And there are cheaper ways to keep an infant's feet warm. The only other thing shoes will do for an infant who is not yet walking, particularly if the shoes are ill-fitting, is harm the feet. So unless you are really anxious to get that first pair of shoes bronzed, I would advise you to save your money until your baby actually needs footwear to protect his or her feet. You don't put glasses on an infant to insure that their eyes develop properly, so why shoes?

I also advise parents not to waste time if they think their infant has a foot problem. If they suspect that their baby has a foot deformity or even a lesser problem, parents are well advised to seek an opinion from a podiatrist or orthopedic surgeon who specializes in children's foot disorders. Conservative treatment of the usual range of infantile foot disorders has a very high success rate if the problem is identified and dealt with at the outset, before the abnormality has had a chance to develop further.

The Club Foot

The number-one fear that expectant parents have about their baby's feet is of a club-foot deformity. A *club foot* is usually twisted downward and inward, although there are variations in which it is twisted outward *(talipes valgus)* or in which just the sole of the foot is turned inward *(talipes varus)*. Unless such a birth defect is corrected immediately, the baby will have a tough time walking normally when it begins trying to get up off all fours.

The club foot is a birth defect that was once thought to be caused by the fetus's abnormal position in the womb during the gestation period. This theory held that there was no particular reason why normal development of the lower limbs was affected during pregnancy; the unborn child just happened to be in the wrong place for too long a time, and the foot did not have space in the womb to grow in the proper direction. However, according to the most recent medical literature on the subject, the position of the fetus in the womb has little to do with the development of a club foot. The literature holds that the ankle bone develops abnormally, causing a dislocation between it and the navicular, which in turn creates further bone and soft-tissue problems during development of the fetus.

A club foot is easily recognizable at birth, so there is no reason to delay treatment. The treatment of choice in mild cases is to place the offending foot and lower leg in a plaster cast, forcing the limb to assume a more normal position. To ensure proper development as the infant grows, the cast is either changed or "wedged" every couple of weeks. A wedged cast has a pie-shaped inversion cut out of it to provide extra space in which the rapidly developing lower limb can grow. When this treatment is initiated immediately upon discovery of the condition, there is little need for more radical steps down the road, and the infant's foot should eventually develop well within normal limits. According to many orthopaedists, in moderate to severe club-foot deformities the treatment ought to be corrective surgery, performed early in infancy to prevent greater abnormal development. After having seen some excellent results, I am inclined to agree with them.

In milder cases, the limb will be in a cast from ten to twenty-six weeks, depending on the severity of the club foot. Thus the shape of the foot ought to be within acceptable limits long before the infant is ready to take his or her first steps.

After the cast has been removed, it is important that complete X-ray evaluation and other follow-up examinations be conducted on a regular basis to ensure that all the bones of the foot and lower leg are present and are growing in the right directions. These follow-up examinations should be conducted for the first two years of the child's life to make sure there is no regression. It is sometimes necessary during this period to place the child in a straight-lasted shoe, which will help maintain the correction during the further early development of the foot.

Other Congenital Problems

A few concerns do arise as a result of poor positioning of the unborn child in the womb. One of these is called *metatarsus adductus,* which is medicalese for the front part of the foot turning inward at birth. The opposite—outward turning—is also possible, but is far less common. This is a condition involving the metatarsal bones only. If only the first metatarsal is involved, the condition is called *metatarsus primus adductus* or *varus.* As with the club foot, metatarsus adductus is uncommon in newborn babies and is readily treatable, particularly if the condition is dealt with from the beginning of the infant's life.

Both metatarsus adductus and metatarsus primus adductus are easily recognized by the trained eye, although when the conditions are very mild they will not be seen until the child begins to walk. However, mild cases respond well to treatment, even if they are not caught at birth.

If either condition is severe enough, it may be necessary to put the offending foot in a plaster cast for the first few weeks of the baby's life. Thereafter—and in most milder cases—it is advisable, whenever necessary, to fit the infant with reversed straight-lasted shoes fastened together by a Denis Browne bar or a Brachman skate. These contraptions are worn while the child is asleep, and they keep the feet properly positioned at all times. It is also important to remember that orthotics may be required to maintain the correction once it has been achieved. If properly treated during the child's early growth period, both metatarsus adductus and metatarsus primus adductus respond exceptionally well, and the infant will be able to stand and walk normally when the time comes.

Another condition that occasionally crops up with newborn infants, and which causes a lot more concern to parents and ogling grandparents than it merits, is overlapping, or curled, toes. One of the ironies of my profession is that my middle child was born with an overlapping toe. The pediatrician who first examined my daughter was highly amused that a podiatrist could help produce a child with such a condition.

An overlapping toe is not a serious deformity. Many such toes will straighten out by themselves, but a few will have to be taped to adjacent toes for a few months to help them develop correct, permanent alignment. During this time there is no discomfort to the infant, only to the concerned family and friends. By the time the infant is ready to get up on its feet, the offending toe, or toes, will have straightened out, and first steps will be just normally awkward, rather than abnormally awkward.

One deformity that is not caused by poor positioning of the fetus in the womb is a condition known as *supernumerary toes,* which is congenital. In this condition, for some reason the developing fetus develops more than five toes per foot. In rare cases a newborn baby has had more than six toes, but I have never seen such a case.

Supernumerary toes can occur on one foot or both feet. Obviously this is one of the easiest disorders to diagnose; the extra toe is usually found on the outside of either the big toe or the baby toe. Not only is the diagnosis simple, but treatment is also relatively easy. The extra toe (or toes) can be removed surgically, either immediately after birth or once the baby is considered strong enough for the operation. A quick fix is not essential for the development of a normal foot, although surgery should be performed as soon as possible and before the baby first attempts to walk. When parents and grandparents become obsessed with their offspring's abnormality, an early resolution to the problem is usually recommended. In any event, surgery is almost always easy and successful. Perhaps parents of children born with extra toes should consider it an omen of extra good fortune, rather than one of bad luck.

Finally, less than 1 percent of all newborn babies arrive on the scene with webbed feet. Contrary to what one might think, this difference does not mean that these children are ugly ducklings doomed to a childhood of woe. During the maturation process in the womb, the toes of the fetus are somehow joined together by skin between the interspaces. As with many minor infant foot problems, it is the parents or grandparents who clamor for immediate surgery. In actual fact, unless X rays show a bone deformity of some sort, there is no reason ever to detach the joined toes. A child can grow up with attached toes and walk or run quite normally, except when they are completely webbed down to the toenails. I have seen quite a few adults with webbed feet who have never experienced any dysfunction or discomfort.

However, some parents insist that their baby be relieved of the webs at once. Fortunately, the procedure is quite simple: minor plastic surgery to cut the skin between the toes followed by stitching of the flaps. The infant will experience little real discomfort, and the incisions should heal quickly.

Now that we have covered the most common lower-limb deformities in infants at birth, let us turn our attention to babies beginning to walk.

The Sneaker Generation

I know it may not be quite as appealing to bronze baby's first pair of sneakers for posterity, but that is the type of footwear your offspring ought to be wearing as they grow up, because sneakers provide the best support for the normal growing foot at the most reasonable cost. Before I explain why sneakers are the preferred form of footwear for the growing child, I would like to trace the development of the foot from the time the child begins to walk until he or she is fully grown.

The first thing to get straight is the fact that a child's limbs do not necessarily grow the same amount at the same time. However, by the end of a youngster's physical development, both legs ought to be the same basic length, give or take a couple of millimeters. So you need not panic if your growing child is listing as he or she walks and you discover that one leg is a bit shorter than the other.

I have seen cases in which children were prescribed lifts for their shoes because at one given moment one leg was longer than the other, and once the lower limbs were both fully grown, the result was a biomechanical problem that would never have occurred otherwise. The moral of the story is not to try to fool with nature; once it has made adjustments for an artificially produced abnormality, those adjustments will be difficult to eliminate completely without further—and expensive—treatment. It is only in rare cases, where the discrepancy in the length of the child's legs is more than one-half to three-quarters of an inch, that parents ought to consider eliminating the difference with special treatment, such as a shoe lift. And it is important even then to watch the child's development carefully so that the lifts can be changed or removed completely as the child grows and leg lengths equalize.

Parents are often unnecessarily concerned if their child is a very late walker. (However, when they realize how much mischief an infant who is walking can get into, as compared to one who is still on all fours, they are sometimes sorry the kid ever took that first step.) Babies usually begin to walk between the ages of ten and eighteen months. Some take their first steps before this if they have developed early physically and their lower limbs can support them; others wait until they are well over two years of age. Often the late starters are not physically ready to walk, but occasionally they simply do not feel the need.

Chapter 8: Children's Feet

In-Toeing and Out-Toeing

When parents come into my office with youngsters who have just begun to walk, their most common complaints are that their offspring are either waddling like ducks or taking pigeon-toed steps. Usually these unusual gaits result from the infant's attempt to maintain balance on still unsteady lower limbs, and the child will begin to walk properly as the lower limbs develop normally. It is common for newly walking babies to toe out dramatically and also to appear to lack arches altogether. These apparent abnormalities in gait are only nature's way of helping the infant balance properly in order to remain erect.

However, if a small child continues to either toe in or toe out, there is probably a bone deformity or muscle weakness in the lower limbs, and the abnormality may have to be corrected. Otherwise, the child will continue to grow and walk abnormally, and will probably be the butt of cruel jokes at school, at play, and even in the home. A child who is constantly being teased about the way he or she walks will not be a happy child.

Abnormal in-toeing and out-toeing can be spotted in a baby's first steps, and it is often sharp-eyed grandparents who are the first to notice the problem. The majority of children with this problem will toe in.

Mild cases of in-toeing or out-toeing are generally caused by a minor bone deformity or muscle weakness. As with most very mild infant foot disorders, detection at birth is not easy, since the foot is shaped normally. The tilt of the foot will be somewhat abnormal, but this tilt is not usually evident until the baby begins to take steps. My advice to parents who have infants with a mild degree of in-toeing or out-toeing is to leave them alone, because, with time, the situation will generally take care of itself. If it becomes obvious after the infant has been walking for a while that he or she has a serious in-toeing or out-toeing problem, this indicates the presence of a more severe bone deformity or muscle weakness. As the problem gets more severe, the treatment must be more aggressive. Rest assured, however, that with proper conservative care your child will not have to waddle like a duck or toe in like a pigeon forever.

The normal amount of in-toeing or out-toeing is about fifteen degrees. Ninety-five percent of the children I see under the age of four who have in-toeing or out-toeing tendencies are within normal limits, and they will eventually outgrow their problems without intervention of any kind. And, as I mentioned above, it is perfectly normal for the arch to appear flat for the first few months—up to three years old—when the baby begins walking. At this point of development, the arch area is filled with "baby fat" that flattens out and cushions the foot, providing better balance and mobility for the child. As the child grows, the arch should develop normally, but if it does not, you ought to consult a specialist for an appraisal of the situation.

If a child is toeing out to the extent that medical intervention is required, the cause is often a tibia (shinbone) deformity—a condition known as *external tibial torsion*—or a misalignment at the ankle joint. The usual treatment is wearing a Denis Browne bar or a Brachman skate (the same contraptions used to rectify metatarsus adductus, discussed earlier) at bedtime. To realign the foot, the bar or skate is attached with the shoes facing inward. It should not be necessary to keep the child in these appliances nightly for more than a few months. The important thing to watch with this treatment is that you do not overcorrect the deformity; otherwise the child will eventually have to wear the bar or skate at night with the shoes facing in the opposite direction. Many new bracing products on the market today can be used instead of the Denis Browne bar; they are a lot more comfortable and will give the same results.

If, for whatever reason, a child is allowed to develop physically without correction of a definite out-toeing problem, it may be necessary for such an older child to wear orthotic devices for eighteen to twenty-four months to correct the disorder. It should be noted that older children do not respond well to wearing appliances on their feet while they sleep.

In-toeing can be caused by metatarsus adductus or by internal tibial torsion, both of which force the foot to turn to the inside. Children who toe in seem to be perpetually off balance, and they are. It is not easy to walk pigeon-toed and keep your balance, whatever your age.

If in-toeing is caused by internal tibial torsion or metatarsus adductus, the treatment is basically the same as for out-toeing. However, when the Denis Browne bar or the Brachman skate is put on, the shoes are pointed outward rather than inward in order to force the feet to the outside. It may also be necessary to use orthotic devices in the child's shoes for up to two years, depending on the severity of the problem. If the condition is spotted early, the treatment usually works quite well. If the cause is excess femoral antiversion (an inward twisting of the thigh bone), which is usually found in three-to-six-year-olds, the "W" sitting position is recommended whenever possible. This position consists of sitting on the haunches with the feet pointing outwards.

Toe-Walkers

When they begin walking, some toddlers never seem to get their heels down on the ground. They zoom around on tiptoe, oblivious to the fact that they are not walking properly. At first, family and friends may think their unusual gait is amusing, before they realize that the child has a problem.

This problem involves Achilles tendons that are too short. Therefore, when the child begins to walk, they are unable to get their heels down on the ground. The solution is to have the toddler's Achilles tendons stretched by a physiotherapist until they reach a proper length. The sooner the therapy can begin, the quicker and more effective the treatment. It may take a while, but eventually the tendons should assume a proper length and the child will begin walking normally. In rare cases the tendons will not respond to physiotherapy, and more aggressive measures, such as surgery, may be necessary.

Growing Pains: Problems of Older Children

Children can still toe in or toe out past the age of three if their conditions are ignored or subsequently acquired. Treatment of these disorders in older kids is different than for toddlers, because older children tend not to want to lie still at night in Denis Browne bars or Brachman skates. They also do not seem to respond to straight-lasted shoes. So what can we do when suddenly concerned parents come rushing into the office with their decidedly knock-kneed, bow-legged, or severely pronating children?

Unfortunately, a few doctors still believe that a child past the age of about eight will outgrow in-toeing or out-toeing. That rarely happens. These children may have to be fitted with orthotics to help realign the foot and lower leg. Orthotics work amazingly well with this age group, and it is always gratifying when I see a child who first came to me with a severe problem begin to

walk normally after a few months of wearing an orthotic device. Of course, some cases take longer to treat successfully, so if your child has been fitted with orthotic devices and you have yet to see dramatic improvement after a few months, be patient.

Young Bunions

Another pain for children from the ages of about five to fifteen is felt directly in the foot. Many children who abnormally pronate severely and are allowed to continue to do so will eventually wind up with a bunion. There are two schools of thought when it comes to treating a bunion on a child's foot, and both of them unfortunately involve surgery. And there is no quick fix for this condition; even if the pronation problem is corrected, the bunion, once developed, will not magically disappear.

I agree with some of my colleagues who feel that bunion surgery on a still-developing foot could result in damage to the *epiphysis* (growth plate) of the big-toe bone. The growth plate is the growing sector at the end of a bone. During the growth period, the epiphysis is separated from the shaft of the bone by a plate of cartilage. The edge of this plate nearest the shaft progressively converts into bone, while the other edge develops new cartilage. This is how bone lengthens in growing youngsters. When the bones are fully grown, the growth plate ceases to exist. The long-term result of a damaged growth plate could be a serious bone deformity. Therefore, we prefer to delay bunion surgery until the growth plate has completely united with the big-toe bone.

The other school of thought maintains that correction of the big-toe bone ought to be done as quickly as possible, before the child has a fully developed foot. Surgeons who hold this belief argue that they do not touch the growth plate at all. Moreover, the earlier the operation is performed, they say, the less damage there will be to soft tissue around the bony deformity, and the more likely it is that the toe will grow in the right direction.

I believe there is merit in the second argument. However, I still prefer to wait until the growth plate of the big-toe bone has fused with the bone, so that there is no further possibility of damage to the plate.

Breaking Up Is Easy to Do

It is hardly uncommon for active children to fracture bones in their limbs. Fortunately, at a young age they tend to heal quickly—usually within four to eight weeks—if they are properly treated by being put in a cast used to immobilize the fractured bone while it mends.

There is no sense going into detail to describe all the possible fractures a child can suffer in the foot, since most of the bones are vulnerable if traumatized severely. But it is important to recognize the symptoms of a break and to deliver the child to a medical center for X-ray evaluation and immediate

treatment. If the child screams in agony when the injured area of the foot is palpated, and if there is considerable swelling accompanying the pain, the possibility of a fracture has to be considered.

Once the diagnosis has been made and the fractured bone is immobilized, the area must by X-rayed periodically until the orthopedic surgeon or podiatrist is convinced that the bone has healed in proper alignment, and that there has been no damage to its growth plate.

Breaking Down under Stress

Another common orthopedic condition in children is *aseptic necrosis* of an epiphysis (growth plate). This is a noninfectious breakdown of the growth plate of a bone. The generally accepted theory in medical circles is that the condition is caused by trauma to part of the bone while the child is playing hard or engaged in some other strenuous activity. In the foot, the most commonly affected bones are the heel bone, the navicular in the midfoot, and the second metatarsal. Because the condition involves the growth plate, and since the growth plate eventually fuses with the end of its bone as the child reaches the late teens, aseptic necrosis of the epiphysis is strictly a childhood disease.

The first example of aseptic necrosis I will discuss is *Freiberg's disease*. If a child constantly complains of pain under the second metatarsal head, especially during or after strenuous activity, there is a good

Chapter 8: Children's Feet

chance that the growth plate of the metatarsal bone is breaking down. In severe cases, the metatarsal head can almost completely disappear, although with time it usually regenerates by itself. I have, however, seen many cases where the bone remains abnormally shaped throughout the person's life. Even if this happens, though, it would be unusual for the pain to persist after the child has stopped growing. If the area remains painful, I X-ray the bone to ascertain whether or not it is regenerating properly, but I would advise patience rather than aggressive intervention if the condition persists.

Sever's disease affects the heel bone of growing, active children—almost always males—and will last until approximately the age of fourteen. The child will complain of a sharp pain in the back of the heel when he or she is playing or running. As with other forms of aseptic necrosis, there is no need to worry excessively about Sever's disease. Once the growth plate has fused solidly to the heel bone, the pain will disappear for good.

The navicular bone is ship-shaped, as you saw in Figure 1.1 (page 7), and it articulates with the three cuneiform bones in front and with the ankle bone at the back. It is a sturdy part of the anatomy, and is rarely mentioned outside medical circles. However, children can fall victim to aseptic necrosis of its growth plate, and they will complain of pain in the area of the navicular bone. The condition is known as *Kohler's navicular* or *Kohler's disease*.

As I have already mentioned, aseptic necrosis of a growth plate can be confirmed by X rays. The affected area, when viewed from the side, will appear ratty or moth-eaten. Of course, nothing is actually gnawing away at the growth plate. And in all cases, natural healing will take place over a period of time until the growth plate fuses solidly to its bone.

If the pain is severe, orthotics can be used to relieve pressure on the affected areas, and it should be noted that orthotics are particularly effective in treating Freiberg's disease as they offload the pressure on the affected metatarsal, thereby reducing the discomfort and allowing for regeneration of the metatarsal head in most cases. An over-the-counter arch support or heal pads may be somewhat effective in offloading the pressure and lessening the discomfort of Sever's disease and Kohler's disease. However, shoe inserts do not cure these conditions; nature does, with time. Proper footwear will also lessen the symptoms. If the pain is particularly acute after strenuous activity, particularly in the heel area, application of ice can help relieve the inflammation

When a child suffers from aseptic necrosis in the foot, the parents may feel it is necessary to curtail their offspring's physical activities. Such a drastic step is usually not necessary. The child should be allowed to continue his or her activities up to the point where discomfort eclipses pleasure because physical activities will not permanently damage the foot.

Young Maid's Knees

Some young women, usually between the ages of thirteen and eighteen, experience annoying knee pain, particularly when going up or down stairs, when getting up after sitting a long time, and intermittently whenever the knee decides to protest. What exactly is the knee protesting about? Well, the condition is familiar to runners; it is called chondromalacia of the patella (kneecap), or "runner's knee," and is discussed in detail in Chapter 11.

Chondromalacia is medicalese for softening of the cartilage in a joint, in this case the kneecap. In young women it is caused by a combination of effects. One theory holds that as the female body develops, the hips spread. The tendons and other soft tissues around the knee do not grow quickly enough to keep up with overall body growth, so a tightness develops, particularly in the patellar tendon. As the pelvic area spreads, the thigh bones take on a different angle relative to the lower limbs. At the same time, a new interest in footwear fashion leads to wearing the wrong shoes. If the young woman has an overpronation syndrome, chondromalacia becomes even more likely.

The second theory holds that the tendons are actually loose and lax, and therefore the patella is pulled to the outside of the knee when it is fully bent. I believe that both theories are true, as I have seen very convincing arguments on both sides.

The overall result of these effects is that the patella is not properly grooved in the knee joint. The knee is being pulled to the inside and the entire leg is rotating internally, basically because of spreading pubescent hips and slow tendon and other soft-tissue development. Dr. Hamilton Hall, an eminent orthopedic surgeon, descriptively calls the end result "teenaged female knee-pain syndrome."

In most cases the treatment for this annoying condition is patience, accompanied by specific muscle-strengthening exercises to take pressure off the knee joint. Orthotics may be required to correct overpronation and to properly align the foot with the knee. It is also necessary for teenage girls with the condition to wear proper footwear—preferably good running shoes, and definitely not high heels.

Only in rare cases, when conservative treatment and time fail to eliminate debilitating pain, will surgery to repair the cartilage damage be required. I would certainly recommend seeking a second opinion if surgery is advised for a young woman's chondromalacia before other, noninvasive measures have been attempted. With the right exercise program and proper footwear, a teenaged female with chondromalacia of the patella ought to have outgrown the disorder by the time she finishes high school.

I have not discussed the foot problems of adolescents in any great detail because most disorders will have been noticed and dealt with before a child reaches fifth grade. Also, once children

Chapter 8: Children's Feet

enter the teenage years, their problems become similar to those of adults—except for cases of aseptic necrosis of the growth plate of a bone—and are discussed in detail in other chapters.

The important thing to remember is that children cannot, or will not, always tell you when their feet hurt; therefore parents have to be very observant of the way their offspring walk and run. And, if a problem does arise, parents must have it taken care of quickly so that the child avoids suffering later and is not required to undergo more aggressive treatments. Finally, and I feel this is worth repeating, parents should not be frightened when a child is born with or develops an abnormality of the lower limbs. If the condition is caught early, non-surgical treatment is usually the norm, not the exception, and your child will not be exposed to lengthy periods of uncomfortable, debilitating convalescence.

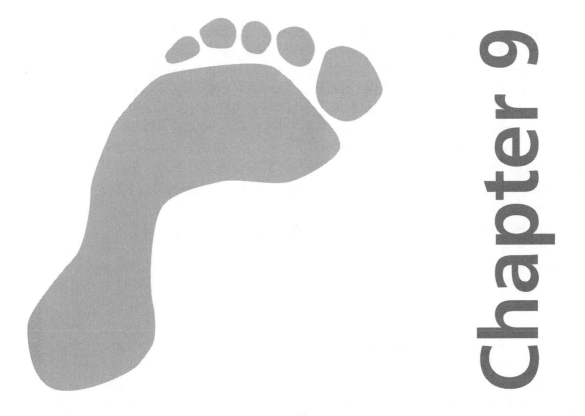

Chapter 9

Geriatric Feet

The early baby boomers, who were born just after the end of the Second World War, are slowly approaching their "golden years." They are also beginning to understand that many of the fitness regimens they have been following to delay the aging process have actually contributed to premature wear and tear on certain parts of their bodies—particularly the joints in their lower extremities, from the lower back to the toes. This is most unfortunate, because exercise done properly will undoubtedly improve quality of life, and perhaps even longevity. But it is difficult to do any type of exercise when you awaken in the morning with painful joints and aching muscles.

I have one female patient in her mid-fifties who a few months ago began to train for a marathon run, despite my protestations that her body type was not conducive to long-distance running. A few weeks ago she attempted a sixteen-mile run, which she heroically completed. Since then she has hardly been able to exercise at all, because one knee hurts too much, one ankle continues to swell during vigorous activity, and she has developed plantar fasciitis in one heel.

"There are greyhounds and chihuahuas," I told her in vain, "and you are not a greyhound." I advised her to run no more than three miles three times a week and, if she wished, to do other forms of exercise on the other days. If she continues on her destructive path, she will be setting herself up for a myriad of arthritic conditions, and perhaps even a stress fracture or two.

Then she will reach her so-called golden years with rusty joints that won't allow her to walk normally, let alone exercise.

So if you want to exercise and still be able to function normally into your old age, pay close attention to Chapter 11 on athletes' feet, and read the following discussion about how to stay out of trouble once you reach retirement age.

The Geriathlete

There is no reason for healthy seniors to abstain from physical activity. That said, although some exceptional senior athletes can run marathons or ski like a teenager, moderation and common sense are the key words to keep in mind. Also, seniors who have not regularly exercised in the years leading up to retirement must have a rigorous physical examination before undertaking any strenuous activities, particularly if they are overweight, have high blood pressure or high cholesterol, and/or have been heavy smokers or drinkers. Those who are deemed up to the task might then want to consult with or hire a qualified athletic trainer to help them set up a sensible exercise program designed to fit their needs. Too many unfit seniors decide to start a vigorous exercise program on their own. I hate to be blunt about this, but they run the risk of dropping dead in their tracks because their pulmonary-cardiovascular system is unable to cope with the sudden strenuous activity, or they may injure themselves so seriously that subsequently, either voluntarily or by necessity, they give up physical activity for the rest of their lives.

As an activity for seniors, my first choice is walking. The speed and distance can be adjusted according to your fitness level. With the exception of swimming, walking causes less wear and tear on the lower extremities than almost all other forms of exercise. For those who hate walking, I recommend activities such as tai chi, Pilates, or even certain types of yoga.

Walking is an excellent form of cardiovascular activity; it can be done anywhere, any time, alone or with others. There are no expensive clubs to join and no schedules to follow. All you need is appropriate clothing and good running shoes (which are better than "walking" shoes). If it is raining or snowing, you can join all those other seniors who walk the corridors of apartment buildings and shopping malls.

Whatever regimen you undertake, listen to what your body is telling you—before all you hear are cries of pain and suffering. If you are hurting, stop or slow down; find out what is causing the pain. A seventy-year-old body cannot withstand physical punishment as well as a Generation X body. Muscles take longer to rebound from strenuous activity; joints may be unable to tolerate the stresses placed upon them. Seniors who suffer from osteoporosis have more brittle bones that can break if overstressed.

Proper footwear is essential for all geriathletes, and many may require orthotics or extra cushioning in their shoes

to prevent foot abnormalities from becoming serious problems. Although walking shoes may look more stylish, I prefer running shoes because they provide more stability and cushioning.

Another issue is socks. Let's face it: As people age their skin becomes less tolerant of stresses on the feet—irritations, inflammations, blistering. Another concern is that seniors often have reduced circulation in their lower extremities, which means that they take longer to recover from a foot ailment or injury because the insufficient blood supply makes it so fewer healing nutrients reach the area. This is one condition Botox can't help! A simple way to prevent or reduce these concerns is to wear proper socks, particularly when exercising. Natural fibers—for example, wool and cotton—absorb moisture, such as perspiration, much better than synthetic fibers. Sweat that is not absorbed will leave feet moist, and thus they can become a haven for fungal infections and other nasty irritations.

Osteoarthritis

There is good and bad news when it comes to osteoarthritis. First the bad: The longer you wait to deal with the problem, the harder it is to treat and the more likely it is that you will settle into a sedentary lifestyle that may lead to added osteoarthritis and other, more serious ailments.

The good news is that prompt, correct treatment can prevent osteoarthritis from worsening, and may even reverse its progress. Moderate exercise may actually help in regeneration of cartilage and synovial fluid in an affected joint. Moreover, there is some evidence that proper exercise may slow or even prevent the onset of osteoporosis, a condition prevalent in postmenopausal women (and some men) that results in extremely brittle bones.

One of the most common sites of osteoarthritis in seniors is the medial compartment of the knee (see Figure 11.3, on page 142). A person who is even slightly bowlegged will place excess weight on the inside (medial) part of the knee. Over the years, the increased stress will erode the cartilage at that part of the knee joint and the bowleggedness will increase, setting up a vicious cycle that wears down the cartilage even more. As the pain increases, the senior becomes more sedentary, often gaining weight, which also increases the stress on the medial compartment of the knee. This is why knee replacements have become so commonplace in North America. However, if the problem is treated early and correctly with orthotics, specially designed exercise programs, and weight loss if necessary, there is hope for people with medial-compartment osteoarthritis.

Hung on the Nail

Seniors often have trouble bending over to examine and care for their feet. This is unfortunate, because many toenail problems develop and flourish sight unseen until they start to hurt. I discuss the major nail problems in Chapter 14, but I wish to stress here that most of the toenail maladies affect seniors in spades. It's just another unfortunate part of the aging process, and the problems are often exacerbated by poor circulation and loss of nerve sensitivity.

If you want to avoid unsightly, painful, diseased toenails, and you are unable to see or care for your feet yourself, you must have them examined regularly by a foot specialist—either a podiatrist or a chiropodist—who will check for infections or inflammations and trim the nails properly.

Drying Out

Another painful reminder as we age is that our skin gets drier. Dry skin on the feet, particularly the heels, can crack and become quite sore. The affected areas can also be more susceptible to inflammation and infections. If an infection occurs, a geriatric with diabetes can develop a very serious problem. So prevention is the key word, and it lies in simple moisturizing creams, particularly those containing vitamin E. These creams need not be expensive, and the only potential side effect is an allergy to the product you buy. Read labels carefully before making a purchase.

Fat Is Fit

At least one foot condition is age specific. The ball of the foot is where the heads of the metatarsal bones are joined to the base of the toe bones. If you examine the ball of an infant's foot you will find a big wad of fat, which is there to protect developing bones from being injured. As the child begins to walk, this fat pad diminishes sufficiently to allow for balance. After that, the fat pad slowly thins as we progress through youth and adulthood to old age. Certain diseases, such as rheumatoid arthritis and diabetes, may cause the pad to thin out more quickly.

During the twentieth century people began to live longer, and hence thinning fat pads became more prevalent. If you live long enough, they may disappear altogether. When this happens, seniors will cry out that their feet seem to be on the verge of bursting through their skin. The skin is dense enough to prevent that, but for these people walking can be excruciatingly painful; the bones of the balls of their feet are being directly exposed to immense pressure every time they bear weight—that is, with every stride. There is nothing left to cushion the bones from this constant pounding, and the area becomes severely inflamed. The pain is further enhanced because the nerve endings on the bottoms of the feet are very close to the surface of the skin.

The least invasive and most logical approach to relieving this unbearable pain is to use cushioning inserts or cushioned running shoes that protect the ball of the foot from excessive weight-bearing stress. A knowledgeable athletic-shoe salesperson will know which shoes and/or inserts best suit your needs. Sometimes I also recommend custom-made orthotics to provide proper weight distribution when the foot is on the ground.

In the rare case where running shoes or cushioning inserts don't do the trick, there is a more invasive treatment. This involves injection of medical-grade collagen into the affected area of the foot. The collagen acts as a replacement for the fat pad. Unfortunately, the collagen usually breaks down after six to twelve months, so it must be reinjected regularly. If you are not squeamish about needles and don't want to wear running shoes, you might consider the collagen option.

A Geriatric Footnote

I hope that all seniors who read this chapter and who are sufficiently healthy to undertake a sensible exercise program will understand that there is no need for them to become couch potatoes after they reach retirement age. Over the years, many of my older patients have lived (and are still living) very active lives, with few arthritic or other problems that affect the lower extremities. They pay close attention to their feet, which helps them avoid—or at least alleviate—some of the pain caused by a number of the conditions I have described. For example, my coauthor's brother is seventy-one years old. He has been running for about thirty years and completed a marathon when he was forty-five. He now runs about five miles four or five times a week, and he has never had an arthritic or serious foot problem. Good genes? Perhaps. But he listened to his body when it told him to ease up on his regimen, and on those days when it tells him to rest, he still listens.

So be smart! There is no reason to be a sedentary senior, as long as you exercise properly. As for you foolish baby boomers who refuse to treat your body with the proper respect, you will probably soon be making an appointment with either a foot specialist or an orthopedic surgeon.

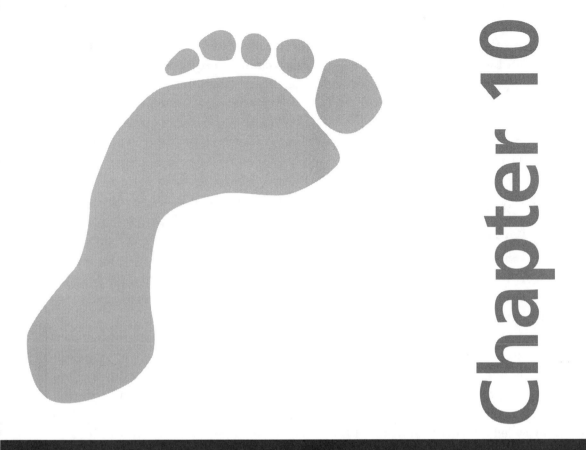

Systemic
Disorders

Chapter 10: Systemic Disorders

Most foot problems are fortunately not systemic, but biomechanical, often resulting from simple wear and tear on the lower extremities. However, everybody is susceptible to a wide variety of systemic disorders, and these diseases can either directly or indirectly affect the feet.

Out of Circulation

My major concern for patients who could develop systemic foot disorders is poor circulation in the lower limbs. Although I routinely check circulation in a patient's feet, I am particularly careful when that patient is older, a smoker, out of shape and/or obese, a diabetic, an alcoholic, or any combination of the above.

As far as I am concerned, one of the major detriments to the health of citizens in the so-called advanced countries of the world is poor nutrition. It has been suggested in clinical literature that a high-fat diet can result in high cholesterol levels in the blood, and that this, in turn, can translate into cardiovascular disease. Cholesterol and other fatty acids will clog arteries as *plaque,* which coats the artery walls and thus narrows the canal through which blood passes. This disease process is called *atherosclerosis.* When it occurs, there is not enough blood flow to certain areas of the body, particularly the outer extremities, since they are farthest from the heart and thus from the place from which fresh, oxygenated blood sets out to nourish the body. Because the foot is farthest from the heart, atherosclerotic symptoms will most likely show up first in the feet and lower legs. These symptoms can be quite varied.

With reduced blood flow to any part of the body, the muscles and tissues may become oxygen-deficient. This causes a condition known as *intermittent claudication,* a disorder that produces a cramping pain—normally induced by exercise—resulting from an inadequate supply of oxygen to the affected muscles. Usually it is the muscles in the calf and lower leg that are involved. At the same time, the patient's feet may be cold and it may be difficult to obtain a pulse in the area.

Because exercise—even normal walking—makes the muscles use up more energy than they do when the body is at rest, a person suffering from intermittent claudication will get relief by sitting down and resting until the pain (which can be quite severe) disappears. Many people with this complaint find that rubbing the affected area also helps relieve the pain. In the long run, rather than just seek temporary relief, it is best to attend quickly to the circulatory problem that is causing the cramps.

Of course, not all muscle cramps in the legs should be interpreted as a sign of serious cardiovascular disease. However, if you develop symptoms of intermittent claudication and your lifestyle or hereditary predisposition points to potential circulatory disease, you would be wise to seek medical advice immediately.

A person with a circulatory problem in the feet may also develop thick and brittle toenails. Hair growth on the lower leg and foot may cease almost completely, and the feet may lose much of their feeling because of damage to nerves in the area. People with circulatory problems are therefore far more prone than the average individual to frostbite, because they are unable to tell when their feet are too cold. Moreover, poor blood circulation to the feet results in insufficient nourishment to the soft tissues and bones, which thus leads to a greater susceptibility to damage from extreme cold or extreme heat.

In severe cases of circulatory disease, the skin on the foot and lower leg may ulcerate because of a serious lack of nutrition to the skin. Unhealthy skin is particularly prone to bacterial infection; poor blood flow to this skin means that bacteria-fighting white blood cells will be unavailable in sufficient quantities to ward off and destroy bacteria at the site of the infection. Nor will the tissue be replenished with oxygen-rich blood. Ulcers develop and the infection becomes even more acute, particularly when a weight-bearing surface of the foot is involved. It is most difficult to treat an ulcerous infection when circulation to the area is impaired, but it is doubly difficult when the wound is continually traumatized by the weight of the body landing on it. There may be, in addition, an impairment to the nervous system called *neuropathy*, which is usually related to diabetes or alcoholism. Since there is decreased sensitivity in the foot, the sufferer may not even feel the damage being done (this will be explained in the next section).

Fortunately, new treatments are available to help check and prevent the severe spread of foot ulcers. These treatments include topical medications, surgical procedures, and even oxygen chambers. Debriding (cleansing) agents are used to clean the open wounds by removing foreign material and dead tissue from the area, thereby facilitating the healing process. It is amazing that, not so many years ago, leg and foot ulcers were often incurable, yet it is equally discomforting that these ulcers are still a common sight, particularly in significantly older people who are not receiving proper medical attention. However, although modern treatment methods have achieved positive results, the best cure for ulcerated feet and legs is still prevention. I strongly urge people with circulatory problems to insist that their feet be regularly examined so that any potentially debilitating problems can be avoided.

The Diabetic Foot

One disease so often associated with circulatory problems in the lower extremities is diabetes. Although this book deals specifically with feet and the lower legs, I should explain a little about diabetes so that you can understand how the condition can adversely affect your feet.

First, here are a few disturbing facts. There are approximately sixteen million diabetics in North America, many of them undiagnosed, and this condition predisposes people to serious ailments of the lower limbs. About 20 percent of diabetics will develop potentially dangerous foot ulcers, and 20 percent of those with foot ulcers will eventually require toe and/or limb amputations in order to survive.

When I refer to sugar in the bloodstream, I am speaking of *glucose,* which is the single source of energy for the human brain and a vital source of nutrition for the rest of the body. There are basically two types of diabetes. In the first type (type 1), the pancreas produces insufficient insulin, which is required to allow sugar to pass from the bloodstream into the cells of the body. This type of diabetes was previously called *juvenile diabetes.* The second form is called mature-onset, adult-onset, or type-2 diabetes, and is more common in adults. In this type of diabetes, the cells become unable to accept insulin, even though the pancreas is producing it in normal, or even increased, amounts. The body is actually resistant to the insulin itself. When this happens, the sugar (glucose) levels in the blood increase while the cells in the body are being starved of their energy source.

Even today, diabetes can only be controlled as it has yet to be cured. And because the disease is always present in the diabetic person, it must be treated with the greatest respect. Often, when the disease is under control, the diabetic thinks he or she has been cured and abandons the regimen that keeps the lid on the disease.

Diabetics can have foot problems for two major reasons, neither of which has yet been fully explained to the satisfaction of medical researchers. The two reasons are neuropathic (affecting the nerves) and circulatory.

Diabetics appear to have a higher percentage of circulatory disorders than the nondiabetic population. Moreover, diabetics who fail to take proper precautions to control their illness are at even greater risk than those who follow a strict regimen of diet and medication. As we discussed above, circulatory disorders often manifest themselves first in the feet, because the lower extremities are farther from the heart than any other part of the body. Therefore, it is vital for all diabetics to be aware of how the disease can affect their feet and how they can avoid serious foot problems. I outline a prevention program on the following pages.

When it relates to the foot, diabetic neuropathy is as dangerous as circulatory disease, and often these two disorders join forces to make life miserable for the diabetic person. At this point we have only theories to attempt to explain why diabetes carries with it the side effect of decreased nerve function.

Because the nerves in the feet are affected, it is often difficult for a diabetic to sense pain or other discomfort, or to distinguish extremely hot and cold temperatures. When poor circulation is combined with loss of sensitivity, the result can be an injury or infection that develops unnoticed until the person is in such dire straits that he or she cannot help noticing the condition. A diabetic may develop a simple blister on a weight-bearing surface of the foot that may turn into an ulcerated lesion that will be extremely difficult to treat and heal. Ulcers can also develop beneath calluses, corns, and ingrown toenails. An ingrown nail can become gangrenous (that is, the tissues in the area die), which may lead to amputation. I do not wish to scare anybody unduly, but I cannot stress too strongly the acute complications that can arise from neglect of a foot infection in a diabetic person.

Because a diabetic—or any other person with a circulatory and/or nerve disorder—can acquire a dangerous infection in the foot without feeling any discomfort, prevention becomes paramount. The list of preventive measures that follows will help you avoid having to deal with such a serious infection:

- Use a file to trim your toenails if you are unable to get them cut professionally. Do not use any sharp object that can cut your foot. And it stands to reason that bathroom surgery of any kind is strictly forbidden!

- Do not wear tight, ill-fitting shoes that can irritate your feet to the point of inflaming them. Some ill-fitting shoes may even cut into your feet and cause the area to become infected. If you have purchased a new pair of shoes, check your feet regularly for the first few days to ensure that they are not causing any damage.

- Check your feet daily, or if you are unable to, have someone else look at them to ensure that no fungal or bacterial infections have erupted.

- Wear natural-fiber—preferably cotton—socks, because they absorb moisture. Dry feet are less prone to infection and inflammation. Do not wear tight, elasticized socks that will hinder circulation in the lower leg and foot.

- Before you step into the bathtub, check the temperature with the back of your hand to ensure that the water is not too hot. If you have reduced nerve function in your feet, you may be unable to judge the temperature with your toes. Scalded feet do not heal quickly.

- As a precautionary measure, you may want to wear support hose to help prevent further damage and, in fact, to assist venous function in the legs. This applies to all people with circulatory problems. Because of poorly functioning veins, feet and ankles swell and become uncomfortable, particularly since shoes no longer fit comfortably. However, do not confuse support hose with tight stockings. Support hose will aid circulation in the lower limbs; tight socks will reduce circulation. Naturally, support hose that are too tight for you will not be beneficial.

- Exercise. Diabetics who exercise are better able to control their condition than those who lead a sedentary lifestyle. Circulation in the legs and feet definitely seems to be better in diabetics who exercise regularly. This may be because of an increase in *collateral circulation,* a phenomenon whereby smaller blood vessels enlarge as bigger ones in the area become clogged. The newly enlarged vessels may then take over some of the circulatory workload and keep the muscles and other parts of the foot energized. Collateral circulation seems to develop more frequently, and with better results, in people who are active. This is nature's way of rerouting traffic away from clogged arteries and onto the side streets. Quite a few medical experts may refute these theories, but some suggest that exercise done properly, combined with the right diet, may even reverse clogging of the arteries.

So I am advising those of you who are diabetic and/or who have circulatory conditions to consult the proper medical specialist about undertaking an exercise program tailored to your physical condition and needs. You need not start running or join an aerobics class; a brisk walk every day will suffice for those unable to do more strenuous exercises. I must emphasize that it is never too late for a diabetic to undertake a proper walking program, even if at first you suffer from intermittent claudication, or muscle cramps in the lower legs. I suspect that these walks will increase your collateral circulation so much that the cramps will eventually disappear. But please, see your doctor first!

- It is a good idea to soak your feet daily in lukewarm water and then apply a moisturizing cream. The daily dunking will help keep your feet clean, and they will therefore be less prone to infection. The cream will keep your skin from becoming dry and cracked, and therefore less prone to infection and inflammation. This daily routine will also force you to look at and touch your feet. Regular examination will help prevent any nasty conditions from establishing a stronghold that will make them more difficult to eradicate than they would have been if quick action were taken.

Gout: The Acid Test

Another systemic disorder that affects the foot—in this case, the big-toe joint—is gout (in medicalese, *podagra,* when it refers specifically to the foot). The big toe seems to be most susceptible, since it is the largest joint in the forefoot and the farthest from the heart. This means that the circulatory system is less able to remove impurities from this joint than from others. In the case of gout, what collects in the joint is uric acid, in the form of crystals. We now know that other crystals also lodge themselves in the big-toe joint, particularly calcium, which is responsible for the development of *pseudo-gout,* an inflammation that mimics gout. When these crystals settle in joints, they can produce excruciating pain that is often mistaken for osteoarthritis.

Gout is often considered to be a disease of the rich, because in the past only wealthy people were able to afford tasty diets rich in fatty foods. However, it now appears that while a "rich" diet will exacerbate a gouty condition, the initial problem lies with the body's inability to properly break down uric acid in the blood. Researchers have theorized that uric acid is not totally useless to the body, and may, in fact, aid the body's immune and endocrine systems. So we no longer identify the typical gouty individual as a man of means, sitting at a fully laden dinner table with grease dripping down onto his royal robes, resting one foot with a hugely swollen big toe gingerly on a stool beside his chair.

The onset of an attack of gout can be sudden and vicious. It is not uncommon for the victim to be awakened in the middle of the night by excruciating pain in the big-toe joint. This terrible, unexpected pain distinguishes gouty arthritis from any other form of arthritis. Osteoarthritis, the most common type by far, is characterized by a much slower onset, chronic pain, and a worsening of discomfort after walking or running. Yet, despite the differences, it never ceases to amaze me how often the two conditions are misdiagnosed. Actually, in most cases a simple blood test to measure the amount of uric acid in the blood will determine whether the patient has gout.

If gout is not treated properly, it will eventually cause permanent changes in the big-toe joint, and the subsequent wear and tear may necessitate some form of invasive treatment. Fortunately, there is no need for the disease ever to progress to that stage. Once the existence of gout has been confirmed, drugs can be prescribed that will control uric acid levels in the blood. Also, if the discomfort is severe, oral nonsteroidal anti-inflammatory drugs can be taken to relieve inflammation in the joint. While gout is definitely not a life-threatening disease, it is indeed a painful one. However, there is absolutely no need for anyone to suffer from gout in this day and age.

Rheumatoid Arthritis

Unfortunately, rheumatoid arthritis is a disease that has yet to be completely tamed. And although it is rarely life-threatening, the relentless pain can at times almost drive people crazy.

Unlike osteoarthritis, rheumatoid arthritis is not brought on by a wear-and-tear process, and it can affect all age groups—I have seen two-year-olds with the disease. It is thought to be an *autoimmune* condition, in which the body's immune system mistakes the joints for foreign matter and tries to destroy them. This is an apparent example of nature functioning at its worst.

Usually all I can do for a patient with rheumatoid arthritis is provide relief for painful joints in the feet and ankles. I will recommend custom-made shoes and soft supplemental inserts to take much of the normal weight off the diseased metatarsal heads.

If you suspect that you may suffer from this disease, a detailed physical examination and blood tests can determine whether or not you actually have it. It is important that this disease be treated by a *rheumatologist,* a specialist well versed in the various diagnostic methods and treatments. Gold injections or cortisone may help alleviate the discomfort, but they do not cure the disease. The same applies for nonsteroidal anti-inflammatory drugs and methotrexate—the present drug of choice for certain patients—taken orally. Modern surgical advances have made total replacement of some joints possible, but this is done only when the distortion of the joint and the pain prevent the patient from functioning with any degree of normalcy. Newer drugs, such as Remicade, which are infused directly into the patient, have been very successful in a number of trials. Unfortunately, this new family of drugs is very expensive and therefore is not readily available to all who might benefit from their use.

Other Systemic Forms of Arthritis

Other forms of arthritis and arthritic-type conditions can also affect the joints of the feet and the lower legs. I have already covered some of them in other chapters; a few are quite rare and are hardly ever seen by foot specialists. Two of those that I do come across from time to time are *psoriatic*

arthritis and *gonococcal arthritis.* I discuss psoriatic arthritis in Chapter 13. Gonococcal arthritis is caused by the spread of gonococcal bacteria into the joints; there is little more I can say about arthritis brought about by an untreated venereal disease. The symptoms are similar to any other type of arthritis, but the treatment is basically the use of antibiotic medication to kill the infection.

Neuromuscular Diseases

It would take a large volume to describe in any detail the various diseases that affect the nerves and/or muscles of the lower limbs. These motor diseases affect the ability of the lower extremities to move normally. But because they are usually diagnosed long before I would get to examine the patient's feet, there is no point in lengthy descriptions that might serve only to unduly worry or confuse the reader. I would be remiss, however, if I did not mention the better-known neuromuscular diseases that affect the feet and legs. However, keep in mind that I am a podiatrist, and therefore not an expert in the diagnosis and treatment of these debilitating disorders.

Until the mid-1950s, when Doctors Salk and Sabin gave the world antipolio vaccines, poliomyelitis was one of the most dreaded of all neuromuscular diseases. Unfortunately, there are still many people limping around today who were unlucky enough to contract polio before it was conquered. They were left with at least partial paralysis in one leg because their motor systems were irreparably damaged.

Polio is now under control around most of the world, but numerous other neuromuscular diseases have to date defied medical researchers. Although these researchers realize that the disorders are caused by a major breakdown of the nervous system, they do not yet understand why the breakdown occurs. As a result, prevention and cures are probably still years away. The diseases we hear about most in this category are multiple sclerosis and amyotrophic lateral sclerosis (ALS, or Lou Gehrig's disease). Both these dreaded diseases eventually rob a person of the ability to use his or her legs and feet.

The Pregnant Foot

Although pregnancy can hardly be classified as a disease, a pregnant woman's system does undergo changes, most of them hormonal. These changes can affect her feet, particularly as she nears her delivery date and is at her heaviest. All this extra weight puts added stress on her feet, especially when she is walking.

When a woman is pregnant, she produces a hormone that causes her ligaments to become fairly lax so that they can expand to provide space for the fetus. All the ligaments expand, not just those in and around her abdomen and pelvic area. As the ligaments in her feet lengthen, her foot naturally becomes wider and flatter. There is good reason for this: The broader, flatter

foot helps distribute the extra weight she is carrying. After a woman delivers, her feet should gradually return to their normal shape, although it is not uncommon for postpartum women to complain that their feet have become permanently enlarged. There is nothing wrong with this situation—as long as the woman buys and wears shoes that fit her new foot size.

I have a bit of advice for pregnant women to help them survive the nine months without having to endure constantly aching feet and legs. First, wear proper footwear! I strongly recommend wearing running shoes with excellent support as often as possible. This type of shoe provides the best shock absorption, and you can loosen the laces when your feet begin to swell over the course of the day.

Second, your feet begin to swell because the veins in your legs empty into your pelvic area, an area that is being cramped by the normal distension of the womb. Because of the traffic jam in the pelvic region, the blood backs up in the veins of the legs and the feet, and they swell. The two best ways to alleviate the situation are to wear properly fitting support hose—remember, not too tight!—and to keep your feet elevated as much as possible.

Finally, if you do have an abnormal pronation problem, it will become more pronounced when you are pregnant because of the change in the shape of your foot. Therefore, you will want to be doubly sure that you control the abnormal pronation during your pregnancy. You will be much more comfortable if you are walking normally, rather than with a biomechanical fault.

Although I advise prevention in almost all cases of biomechanical foot problems, how can I object to motherhood? Yet my mother constantly reminds me that her foot problems began after I was conceived. I try to tell her, as well as all my pregnant patients, that if they follow the advice I give them, they will remain reasonably comfortable while standing and walking, and most likely will have perfectly normal feet within weeks of delivery.

Varicose Veins

It is not abnormal for veins in the legs and feet to perform less than adequately for reasons that have little to do with any specific, serious circulatory condition. That is why I have not lumped this discussion of veins and their problems with other circulatory diseases.

Varicose veins are veins that have valve problems. Veins have valves that open to allow blood to pass through and then close to prevent it from flowing backward. This opening and closing action is designed to return spent blood to the heart for passage to the lungs to be reoxygenated. Unlike the arteries, which carry fresh blood to the various parts of the body, the veins have no muscle fibers to pump the blood. Therefore, the valves are needed to assist the blood in flowing back to the heart. Obesity, pregnancy, and overall poor venous

function can contribute to the malfunctioning of these valves. When this happens, blood begins to back up in the veins because it is no longer being forced upward.

This condition normally affects the superficial veins in the lower leg, particularly on the back or side of the leg. These veins expand because of the blood they are being forced to hold, until eventually they do not function properly. The larger, deeper veins develop valve problems, causing the used blood to reroute through smaller, more superficial veins nearby. These veins are not designed to carry so much blood, and they begin to bulge. People with varicose veins can often be said to suffer from the blues, because the veins usually affected are close to the surface of the skin, and their blue outlines can become quite noticeable. More seriously, while pressure is building up in these veins, people can experience significant pain, often to the point where invasive treatment is required.

People develop varicose veins for a number of reasons, and I have already mentioned a few: obesity, pregnancy, and poor valve function. Some people may be victims of their work environments: Standing in one spot for long hours every day puts tremendous pressure on the legs. As muscles tighten and the areas through which the veins must pass become impeded, the strain affects the circulation. Deoxygenated blood gets backed up in the veins, which can then swell and eventually develop valve problems. (For pregnant women, the problem arises from poor venous function in the pelvic area rather that in the lower legs themselves.)

If you discover that you are developing varicose veins, what can you do to relieve the symptoms and prevent the situation from deteriorating? First, you need to change your work habits as much as possible, so that you are not standing in one spot for long periods of time. Second, you should wear support hose because, as I previously mentioned, they help venous function by putting pressure on the veins so they will not distend as much.

If you have painful and/or unsightly varicose veins and wish to do something to improve them, you could undergo a procedure to remove or collapse the veins. The blood will find its way naturally into veins nearby. Surgery is the choice when the larger veins are involved; *sclerosing,* or chemical destruction of the veins using an injected solution, can be quite effective for tiny "spider" veins.

A Swell Time

Many people complain of swollen feet and ankles when they have been sitting or standing in one place for a long time, particularly in hot, muggy conditions. Unless they have already been diagnosed with a circulatory problem, they should not worry too much, because this is a normal phenomenon.

Because many people complain of this problem during long airplane flights, a misconception has developed that the atmosphere in the plane is the cause. How-

ever, it is actually the sitting position that is to blame. When your legs are bent at the knees, the area in which the blood flows back through the veins is cramped, and the circulatory system in your lower extremities is adversely affected. Normal venous function becomes temporarily disrupted. The obvious solution is to walk around as much as possible during the flight to allow the lower limbs to stretch out and to increase the space through which the veins pass. Or, if you are lucky enough to be on a fairly empty plane, put up your feet and relax. The law of gravity will take care of your legs' venous function.

Demon Rum and Evil Weed

I have seen too many patients who shrink at the thought of "poisoning" themselves with any type of medication, but who think nothing of the toxicity of the cigarettes they smoke or the excessive amounts of alcohol they consume. Although these people are right to be concerned about the potentially dangerous side effects of certain drugs, they ought to be more aware of what excessive alcohol and smoking can do to their systems.

Before we speak of alcohol and tobacco specifically, I must define two terms for you. The first is *vasodilation,* which refers to temporary expansion of a blood vessel. Heat is an example of a vasodilator, as are a number of drugs and other chemicals that we ingest or inject. *Vasoconstriction* is the opposite of vasodilation and can be caused by cold or by a variety of different drugs and chemicals. Tobacco is a well-known vasoconstrictor. Keep in mind, then, that vasodilators work to increase blood flow through the circulatory system, and vasoconstrictors act to decrease blood flow, a decrease that can become acute and/or chronic.

There is little doubt in medical circles today that smoking can not only damage the lungs, but can also contribute greatly to cardiovascular disease, which can affect the feet. I join with cardiovascular specialists in strongly urging my patients with systemic foot conditions to quit smoking. Many vascular surgeons absolutely refuse to operate on patients who will not, or cannot, quit smoking. Naturally, we doctors do not confine our advice to those who are already ill. An ounce of prevention is worth much more than just a pound of cure. Quitting smoking will keep you on your feet, and healthier, for a lot longer than if you continue to puff away.

As for the "demon rum," it is supposedly not that bad for you from a medical standpoint—if consumed in limited amounts. Studies have indicated that small quantities of alcohol may act as vasodilators and can therefore improve blood flow for a couple of hours in people with circulatory problems. A lot has been written lately about the benefits of red wine. I will not expand on this, but I suggest that much new medical literature will be filled with goodies that can be attributed to the magic grape!

On the other hand, consumption of large amounts of alcohol over a long period of time is destructive to the human body, as we all know. Many addictive drinkers first show signs of *alcoholic neuropathy* in their legs and feet. This means that nerve function in their lower limbs has been affected as the cumulative effects of consumption of large quantities of alcohol attack the central nervous system. So if you like to drink and begin to experience pins and needles, numbness, and loss of sensation in your feet, you would be wise to seek a medical opinion at once. You could be on the verge of self-destructing.

Other recreational drugs and medications may adversely affect the lower extremities, but it would take a few volumes to cover all the potential risks. I suggest that if you are at all concerned about the side effects of drugs or other products that you may be ingesting, you ought to consult with your family physician or another qualified expert on the toxicity of such things as medications, recreational drugs, and food additives.

Cold Comfort

Before discussing serious problems like immersion foot (chilblain) and frostbite, I would like to clear up a couple of misconceptions. First, there is absolutely no connection between having so-called cold feet and being afraid to do something. Your extremities do not necessarily drop in temperature when you are fearful about making a major decision. Second, if you get your feet wet, you are no more likely to catch cold than if you were perfectly dry. If you leave your feet sitting in cold water long enough, you may eventually cause some damage to them, but you will not suddenly develop the symptoms of a viral infection.

Immersion foot, or *chilblain,* is probably the most common cold-related injury to affect the feet. It can occur in temperatures from well below freezing to as high as 60°F. A damp environment, particularly a wet shoe, is often a contributing condition. Immersion foot most commonly affects those with poor circulation, particularly women who wear tight-fitting shoes that reduce circulation to the forefoot.

Symptoms of immersion foot include a whitish color in the affected area, some edema (swelling) caused by buildup of protective fluid under the skin, blistering from the edema, itching, and some pain. However, the affected part of the foot is not frozen.

The treatment is relatively uncomplicated. Analgesics may be required for a few days to relieve pain in the affected area. Whirlpool baths may help increase circulation in the feet. A change in footwear may also be necessary. Care must be taken to ensure that blisters do not break and become infected. Because the disorder can recur quite easily in certain environmental conditions, it is advisable to avoid cold, damp weather whenever possible. If you must be out in inclement weather, wear

two pairs of socks to better insulate your feet. Wool socks keep feet warm because they trap the most heat. Silk is not bad, if you can afford it, and certain types of padding and liners can also help keep the feet warm and dry. If you are active outside in cold weather, try not to wear cotton socks, because cotton absorbs too much moisture and dries slowly, and its ability to trap and hold warm air between its fibers is not as good as that of other fabrics.

Frostbite is far more serious than immersion foot. It may be quite superficial and involve only the outermost layers of the skin, or it can penetrate the entire foot to the point where the only treatment is amputation to prevent the spread of gangrene.

In frostbitten areas of the feet, the blood, nerve, and soft-tissue cells are frozen. If the damage is extensive and deep, it may be permanent. Therefore, the utmost caution must be taken to prevent the onset of frostbite and, if it has occurred, to treat it quickly and properly.

The symptoms of frostbite vary somewhat from those of immersion foot. The skin initially becomes bluish-white and there is a burning pain in the affected area. Eventually the skin assumes a waxy appearance and feels warm. But the foot will soon become numb and feel very heavy. There will be occasional tingling sensations, along with the numb, heavy feeling.

The best treatment for any degree of frostbite is immediate medical attention. If that is not possible, there are a few steps to help you avoid and a few you can take to minimize damage to the foot. First, do not rub the affected part of the foot, especially with something cold, like snow. There is no circulation in the frostbitten area, so rubbing it will accomplish nothing, and the cold snow will only increase the insult. Second, do not expose the frostbitten area to extreme heat, such as hot water or a fire, as you may accidentally burn already damaged tissue. Third, do not smoke or drink alcohol, because blood flow to the foot will be further decreased. Fourth, it is probably wise to try not to walk on the affected foot. I say "probably" because some medical researchers do not believe that this precaution is necessary.

I advise that the affected area be soaked immediately in tepid water, although some experts believe that the water may be warmer—but not hot. Once the entire foot becomes reddish in color—after about twenty minutes if the frostbite is not too severe—it may be removed from the water. Pain will probably be acute in the affected area during the thawing-out process, so it might be advisable to take a strong analgesic. To help increase blood flow to the feet, some frostbite experts also recommend that the victim drink warm liquids, or even a *small* amount of alcohol, after the foot has been soaked.

The feet will swell because of a buildup of protective fluid. To reduce the edema, it is prudent to keep the lower extremities as elevated as possible after the frostbitten area has been removed from the warm water.

Frostbitten parts of the body are more susceptible to bacterial infection than normal tissue. They may also be more prone to fungal infection during the recovery process. It would be wise to ensure that these infections never get a chance to develop. To that end, I repeat, it is vital that proper medical attention be received as soon as possible after the injury has occurred.

As you might expect, once a part of the foot has been subjected to frostbite, it will be more vulnerable to repeated episodes than will unaffected areas. So you will have to take certain precautions to prevent recurrence of such an insult. I strongly recommend that proper footwear—including shoes, inserts, and stockings—be worn in cold weather. And, if at all possible, a person who has suffered from frostbite should try to avoid being exposed to extremely cold temperatures.

Raynaud's Syndrome

Raynaud's syndrome, which primarily affects women, occurs in cool or cold weather. For some reason, the cold creates a very strong reaction in the blood vessels feeding the fingers and toes. This causes the vessels to spasm, which can be quite painful—and somewhat serious if the proper precautions aren't taken, because of lack of blood flow to these extremities. Victims may also complain that their fingers go pale or turn blue very quickly when the syndrome attacks them. Most of the time the condition is not cause for alarm, and dressing properly in cool or cold weather can prevent an occurrence. However, there are times when the syndrome is quite severe; it is then called *Raynaud's disease,* and it requires immediate attention. Because Raynaud's can be a symptom of an underlying, more serious disorder, it should always be investigated when it first occurs.

This ends our discussion of foot problems caused by systemic diseases. Please keep in mind that when it comes to podiatric practice, these conditions are the exceptions rather than the norm. I suggest that if you have foot problems that you are concerned may be systemic, you should not hesitate to seek immediate medical attention. It is far better to be reassured by a doctor that the problem is not serious than to wander around wondering if your health is in danger.

Chapter 11

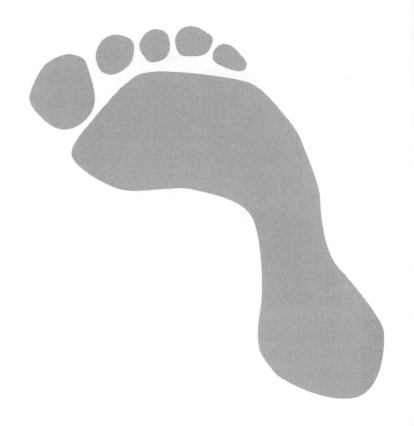

Athletes' Feet I: Runners

Years ago, sports medicine was confined to treatment of injuries suffered by professional or other highly competitive athletes. Those injuries were most often treated by orthopedic surgeons because bones and joints were thought to be the parts of the body most often damaged by contact sports and other demanding activities. If a noncompetitive athlete had a sports-related injury, the usual remedy was a visit to the family doctor, who might prescribe rest, an analgesic, and elimination of strenuous activity for a lengthy period, if not permanently. Fortunately, this is no longer the case, because in North America alone there are millions of adults who exercise regularly in one way or another. Thus, the need arose to broaden the field of sports medicine to treat amateur athletes, who are, of course, just as prone to injury as are professionals.

Many of us associate the initial fitness craze with running or jogging (that is, running slowly). In 1984, a major North American running-shoe manufacturer grossed just under one billion dollars from the sale of its shoes. Now the sports-shoe industry generates annual revenues in the neighborhood of a hundred times that amount, if you include continued sales of running shoes and a whole host of other footwear products, including in-line skates, geared to every conceivable type of athletic endeavor.

Since I last wrote about feet, many other types of physical activity have become popular. The S.C. Cooper Family Sports Medicine Clinic at Mount Sinai Hospital, where I attend regularly, sees thousands of patients a year—people who are involved in a wide variety of exercise regimens, whether on their own or with teams or other groups. Although a number of patients still come in with injuries resulting from racket sports (tennis, squash, racketball, badminton), their visits are nowhere as frequent as they once were. Running has made a comeback, and runners and joggers still make up the largest percentage of the clinic's patient pool. The next largest group includes those involved in a wide range of aerobic activities: cycling, step and low-impact aerobics, working out on machines that simulate cross-country skiing and similar strenuous activities, in-line skating, walking and running on treadmills, and using stair-climbers and elliptical machines. Other popular sports, played either professionally or at the amateur level, also pique the interest of both athletes and spectators, and I will discuss many of them in Chapter 12.

There are different reasons for the popularity of these various activities, not the least of which is the health-conscious person's desire to stay fit. Some people join health clubs both to work out and to socialize; many play certain games to satisfy their competitive personalities. But running is a different matter: runners are often completely uninterested in combining exercise with socializing. They derive their enjoyment from communing with nature and from what is often called a "runner's high," which is thought to result from the body's production of endorphins—one's personal opiate. Apparently, the more you exercise, the more you produce these endorphins; the more endorphins you produce, the less you feel pain and other discomfort and the more you feel a sense of euphoria.

What does all this have to do with feet? Simply that those of us who run, play racket sports, or do aerobics often tend to exercise through our pain-tolerance levels. When we do that, we are setting ourselves up for a sports-related injury. When something hurts, it is nature's way of telling us that something is amiss and that we ought to stop and rest. Often people don't get the message until they are in the middle of exercising or afterwards that some part of their body is not functioning normally, and only then will they seek medical attention. By that time it is often too late to treat the dysfunction easily.

The most common complaints sports medicine doctors see are lower-extremity problems caused by overuse. Approximately 25 percent of patients at most clinics have some sort of knee problem, the same number complain of foot disorders, and about 20 percent of complaints involve the hip and lower back. Another 20 percent involve the neck, shoulders, and elbows—primarily overuse syndromes from too much swimming, weight lifting, and use of exercise equipment. Shin splints used to produce a large number of patients, but since step and low-impact aerobics have in many cases replaced the high-impact type, that injury has become far less common.

A large percentage of knee, leg, and foot problems are directly traceable to poor biomechanics of the lower limbs. The same can also be said for hip and lower-back complaints. This makes me a very busy man, and it is gratifying to watch patients with these disorders improve as a result of our ability to correct biomechanical faults of the feet by using the proper orthotics.

I must emphasize that most of what I am about to say about runners also applies to people who use treadmills or get their exercise by undertaking a serious walking regimen. I treat many of those people for complaints such as metatarsal-head pain, neuromas, plantar fasciitis, and shin splints. It's not a question of how fast you go, but how far, for how long, and in what type of footwear—and, of course, your biomechanics.

I have rarely seen a sight as forlorn as a dedicated runner derailed by an injury. And this is sad, because there is such a wide variety of ailments that can plague a runner—from the toenails all the way up to the spinal column. In fact the miseries are so numerous, I thought it best to break them down according to the parts of the lower limbs and spine that they can affect.

The Black Badge of Courage

Athletes who run long distances, whether at one stretch or over a period of days, can eventually wind up with blackened toenails;

the color comes from blood that has dried and clotted under the nail. What happens is that the longer you run, the more your feet swell from the heat generated inside the shoe. After a while the running shoe becomes too small, and with each step it collides with the front part of the foot, and hence with the toenails.

This friction causes damage to the nail and the nail bed. The nail is rubbed by the shoe, and in turn the nail rubs against the nail bed. Blisters form to protect the area, and the irritation causes some pinpoint bleeding. The blisters may break, and as the fluid from them and from the clotting blood dries, the skin around the area will stick to the nail. The end result is damage to the nail-growing cells, which causes the nails to grow abnormally. If damage to the nail matrix is severe, a runner with the black badge of courage has a discolored, disfigured nail that may never return to normal.

Obviously, this badge of courage can be at least partially avoided. You can simply stop running long distances, or you can take the preventive step of wearing the best-fitting running shoes possible, although this is not always a simple matter under certain conditions or during lengthy runs. Having an extra, larger pair of shoes handy during a long run would be one solution, albeit perhaps not a practical one. Maybe some genius will eventually invent running shoes that automatically expand to fit the constantly swelling foot.

A possible side effect of the black badge of courage is the development of a fungal infection, since the resulting conditions are ideal for the growth of such an infection. If you do develop a discolored toenail, it would be wise to apply an antifungal preparation regularly for the duration of the disorder. If the badge of courage is allowed to develop untreated, the nail may become so badly damaged that it will fall off. This in itself is not a big deal, and the nail will eventually grow back, although its shape may be abnormal. On a positive note, the disorder is more aesthetically unpleasant than it is dysfunctional or uncomfortable, and it is hardly serious enough to prevent you from putting in your daily quota of miles or kilometers.

A Blistering Pace

Athletes are regularly plagued by blisters on parts of their bodies that are subjected to undue friction. As an example, in my many years as podiatric consultant to the Toronto Blue Jays, I have seen many baseball pitchers forced to leave a game because they developed painful finger blisters from gripping the ball extremely hard in order to throw certain pitches, particularly on hot, humid days

Blisters are nature's way of trying to protect the inner layer of skin (dermis) from becoming inflamed. A watery sac develops in the lining between the dermis and the outer layer of skin (epidermis) to prevent inflammatory friction from attacking the inner layer. However, as anyone who has suffered from them knows, the blisters themselves cause severe soreness or pain, particularly if the irritation continues.

Runners develop blisters, and not just under their toenails. The most common areas for blisters on a runner's foot are under the first metatarsal head and on the ends of the toes. These are the areas where the foot is most often subjected to friction caused by overexercising and by wearing poor footwear.

Blisters are easy to diagnose and relatively simple to treat, since the cause of the friction that produced them need only be removed. In most cases, all that is required is a change of footwear. Properly fitting shoes, and stockings or socks that allow the foot to breathe normally ought to prevent most blisters from forming. If, however, the blisters persist, it may be advisable to try a cheap insole to support the arch and prevent the foot from sliding forward. Another technique to prevent blisters is the use of moisturizing creams under a protective bandage. The key here is the thicker the bandage, the less the pressure.

If you continue to run on blistered feet, over a period of weeks a callus will eventually form at the affected area to protect the dermis. This is another example of nature at work. Of course you will then have another problem to deal with, but the blisters will not normally reappear where they flourished before the callus developed.

One problem that can arise with a broken blister is the possibility of infection. It may become necessary to treat a broken blister with an antiseptic and to cover it with some sort of bandage. To relieve pressure, a painful blister may be deliberately broken with a sterile instrument. If this is done, however, care must still be taken to prevent development of an infection.

Heel blisters are far less common in runners. Only poorly fitting shoes and very long runs will cause such a problem. However, in-line skaters often develop heel and lower-leg blisters from wearing skates that don't fit properly.

Fore-Lorn

Runners constantly stress the front part of their feet, and they are therefore very susceptible to forefoot injuries. You will recall from Chapter 4 that the forefoot is the workhorse of the foot, because it is in contact with the ground 75 percent of the time during the stance phase of the gait cycle. It stands to reason, then, that runners, who land harder when striding than walkers, are subjecting their forefoot to even more pounding than the average person does.

Because the forefoot is subjected to such pressure, it is not uncommon for a runner to develop injuries such as metatarsal-head stress fractures (particularly after long runs), neuromas and other nerve-entrapment conditions, capsulitis or synovitis of the metatarso-phalangeal joint, and sesamoiditis or fractured sesamoids.

As I mentioned in Chapter 4, metatarsal stress fractures occur in runners who have subjected their feet to undue stress, such as running too far for too long in the wrong shoes. A runner may hear a *pop* during the run, but will not feel any pain or notice any swelling in the area of the metatarsal head until a few hours later. Then the pain becomes quite noticeable.

I have already discussed the symptoms and treatment of metatarsal stress fractures in Chapter 4, but there are a few points to make here so that runners will not prolong their discomfort. Metatarsal stress fractures will heal by themselves under normal circumstances. Abnormal conditions include trying to run through the injury. The normal recovery time for the fracture is four to six weeks, although it may take older people up to six months to heal completely.

If you run before the fracture has healed, not only will recovery time be longer, but also the pain will linger and be more severe. There is also a distinct possibility that when the bone does eventually heal, you will be left with an abnormality that could eventually cause trouble. So, do not try to be a hero. If you fracture a metatarsal bone, bite the bullet and quit running until the healing process has been completed. A medical expert will advise you when to begin running again and will suggest other activities that you can undertake in the meantime to keep in decent condition.

Talking Horse Sense: Sesamoid Problems

Although fractured sesamoid bones have landed many a horse in the glue factory,

the same fate hardly applies to humans. However, as you learned in Chapter 4, a fractured sesamoid can be troublesome and may have to be removed surgically. If surgery is required, it can be performed on an outpatient basis, and the runner should be able to begin running again in about three to five weeks. The same recovery time is usually indicated for a sesamoid bone that has fractured but does not need to be excised surgically. Once again, the important thing for a runner to remember is that they should not try to run through the injury. Patience is necessary, for the sesamoid bone will rarely heal completely. But do not despair; a person with a fractured sesamoid is often relatively symptom-free once the inflammation from the break has calmed down. The bone remains bipartite (in two pieces) but causes no further problems—in most cases. In all my years of examining feet, I have seen only one sesamoid fracture that healed completely, yet it is the exception rather than the rule to remove the fractured bone surgically.

I discussed chronic sesamoiditis in Chapter 4. It is often more difficult to diagnose the inflammation than the break, and it is just as difficult to treat aggressively because of the constant pounding even normal walking inflicts on an area that is already inflamed. However, the chronic discomfort and swelling can be reduced by ultrasound and ice, and, if deemed advisable by a medical professional, by two cortisone injections given two weeks apart. However, with all these treatments the success rate is at best 50 percent. If the inflammation is acute, the injections or oral nonsteroidal anti-inflammatory drugs may help. If the problem persists, orthotics designed to take weight off the forefoot could be of some value. More than likely, the inflammation will take time to heal, and the runner will have to be patient for a few weeks and, until the discomfort has disappeared, do other exercises that do not stress the forefoot. Women will also have to refrain from wearing high-heeled shoes that put extra pressure on the forefoot.

Nerve-Wracking

Neuromas and other nerve entrapments on top of the foot are not uncommon in runners and other athletes, particularly in-line skaters and cyclists. Unlike the nonathlete, serious runners develop neuromas traumatically, rather than gradually over a period of time. Since the pain is in the general area of the metatarsal head, it is often mistaken for capsulitis or synovitis of the metatarso-phalangeal joint. However, the latter conditions are more often caused by sports activities other than running. If you recall our discussion of these conditions in Chapter 4, you will know that inflammation of the joint can result in impingement of the nerve running between the toes through the affected space. Therefore, it is possible to suffer from a neuroma and from synovitis or capsulitis at the same time.

One of the major causes of forefoot neuromas in runners is running on uneven surfaces for a fairly long period of time and on a continuous basis. For example, if you run five miles a day on a banked surface for a week, you put a tremendous amount of excess stress on the metatarsal heads, because you are creating an artificial overpronation in one foot. In many cities, most roads are banked somewhat to allow for water run-off so that streets will not flood. If you run on the inside part of the road, the foot closest to the curb will be a few degrees lower than the other foot. The artificially induced pronation that results puts extra pressure on the metatarsal heads of the lower foot. If you already have a slight overpronation problem, running on city streets could well increase the risk of a lower-limb injury.

This severe pressure on the metatarsal heads can cause pinching of the nerves in the forefoot, particularly in the areas between the metatarsal bones, near the metatarsal heads. This could result in development of a neuroma. The obvious way to reduce this risk would be to run on as level a surface as possible at all times.

Another potential cause of a forefoot neuroma is wearing running shoes that are too tight, either to begin with or after you have run for a long time and your feet have swelled considerably. Obviously, tight running shoes will force the metatarsal bones to scrunch together, impinging on the nerves passing through the spaces between the bones. The best way to avoid this problem is to ensure that your running shoes fit as perfectly as possible and are not tied too tightly. And if you do have a problem with forefoot neuromas, it would be wise for you to stop running when your shoes start to feel uncomfortably tight.

If a neuroma persists despite a change of running conditions and running shoes, have your podiatrist pad and tape the offending area to separate the metatarsal bones. You should also consider orthotic inserts as a long-term preventive measure to control troublesome neuromas. If the inflammation at the onset of the neuroma is acute, anti-inflammatory drugs or cortisone (if injected outside the joint) may be effective. Surgery to remove the impingement is strictly a last resort.

Calluses, Corns, and Hammer Toes

Runners and in-line skaters get calluses, corns, and hammer toes for the same reason as nonrunners: faulty biomechanics of the feet and lower limbs. Calluses may also develop on the bottom of the foot—particularly under the toes—in response to the need to protect sensitive areas from friction that causes blisters.

The treatment for these conditions is the same for runners as for the general population. The biomechanical fault must be corrected. For runners, this may involve a simple change of running shoes, since almost all modern shoes have built-in supportive devices. However, orthotics may also be necessary. There is certainly no need

for you to give up your favorite pastime just because a callus, corn, or hammer-toe problem persists and has become uncomfortable. With the proper footwear, there is no reason why these conditions cannot be controlled and eventually eliminated. Obviously, a hammer toe might have to be surgically repaired. But assuming the operation is done properly, you ought to be able to resume a running program within a matter of weeks.

Midfoot Crises

I have devoted scant space in this book to the midfoot. That is because, as I have mentioned, very little ever goes wrong with its component parts. However, runners and other athletes can injure the area, particularly the tendons that are attached to the midfoot bones.

Tendonitis (inflammation of the tendons) occurs in runners who have biomechanical faults that create an imbalance in weight distribution on the foot and cause muscles to overstretch. As you learned in earlier chapters, muscles are attached to bones by tendons, and overstretched tendons pull away or are torn away from the bones to which they are attached. The tearing or fraying of the tendons—and the resulting periostitis (inflammation of the lining of the bone)—sets up an inflammation that can be quite painful and may require a lengthy healing period.

The four major antipronation muscles of the foot are the tibialis posterior and tibialis anterior, extensor digitorum longus, and extensor hallucis longus. When a person is not running, a three-degree pronation poses no problem for these muscles. However, when runners are in full flight, they automatically place extra stress on their feet, and even a four-degree pronation becomes excessive, forcing these four muscles to stretch to their limits. As a result, the tendons at the ends of the muscles become prone to fraying or tearing. This situation sets up an inflammation at the spot where the tendons are attached to the bones of the feet.

Tendon sheaths (the coverings of the tendons) generally have a poor supply of blood, so inflamed and torn tendons do not normally heal quickly. As a result, it is not uncommon for a runner who has developed tendonitis in a foot to be advised by the family doctor to give up running for good to allow the tendon to heal and remain healthy and to prevent a recurrence of the problem. If you have been given such advice, you would do well to seek a second opinion from an expert in sports medicine.

Because tendonitis is often so difficult to treat and takes such a long time to heal, the problem ought to be nipped in the bud. Although the major causes of tendonitis in the runner are faulty biomechanics and overuse syndrome (doing too much too soon), it can be brought on and exacerbated by neglecting to warm up and stretch properly—if at all—before beginning to run.

Of course, you may do all the proper exercises and still have tendonitis, caused by a biomechanical fault in your foot that did not cause problems before you began running seriously. Therefore, at the earliest indication of pain in the foot while you are running, it is important that you stop and seek expert advice, particularly from a medical professional specializing in feet and sports medicine.

Once tendonitis has been diagnosed and the cause has been determined to be biomechanical, the obvious next step is to place an orthotic in your running shoe to eliminate the fault—which is usually abnormal pronation. If the tendonitis is acute, you will have to stop running until the inflammation clears up. Anti-inflammatory drugs, ice, and/or ultrasound treatments may help. Once the tendon has healed sufficiently, it would be wise to undertake a proper stretching program to ensure that the muscles and tendons of the foot are in the best possible condition to prevent further trouble. I suggest that you learn the exercises that are best for you from a sports-medicine therapist.

The tendons of other muscles in the foot are also susceptible to inflammation from irritation caused by a runner's foot that is out of sync. The muscles affected in the midfoot area are the extensor hallucis longus and brevis, the flexor hallucis longus and brevis, and the flexor digitorum longus and brevis. They, too, are inflamed by either a biomechanical fault or by an external factor, such as poorly fitting running shoes or running on uneven surfaces. As with other cases of tendonitis, inflammation of the tendons of these six muscles can be identified by pain in the area. Since inflammation of these tendons is so difficult to treat, prevention is obviously the best medicine.

Tendonitis is often referred to today as repetitive strain injury (RSI), which is very common in people who perform the same task over and over again—for example, computer operators, assembly line workers, musicians, and some athletes. Abnormal muscle activity obviously affects the tendons, which can then become overstressed and inflamed. Also, when one set of muscles malfunctions, adjacent muscles try to take up the slack. Eventually the adjacent muscles and their tendons can also become overworked and inflamed, and the pain spreads. Determining which specific muscles and muscle groups are malfunctioning can lead to therapeutic programs designed to get them working properly again.

Plantar Fasciitis

We have already discussed the causes and treatment of plantar fasciitis, one of the most common and least understood foot problems, in Chapter 7. As you will remember, this condition is often referred to as heel spurs, and is named after the spurs that actually form to alleviate the painful situation rather than acting as the cause of it. You will recall that the plantar fasciae are attached to the heel bone and to the five metatarsal bones in the forefoot (see Figure 7.2, page 78). The primary functions of these ligaments are to support the longitudinal arch of the foot and to help control overpronation.

Plantar fasciitis is very common in athletes, particularly those engaged in activities that require constant side-to-side motion—for example, tennis or squash players. The repeated, sudden lateral movements place tremendous torque-like stresses on the entire foot. However, plantar fasciitis has become increasingly prevalent in the general population because of more active adult lifestyles and the wearing of improper footwear, particularly when engaged in wear-and-tear activities. In fact, this condition is very much an overuse syndrome.

The distinctive symptoms of plantar fasciitis are acute pain in the middle and inside rear of the heel, particularly first thing in the morning and after prolonged sitting. There is no discoloration, and swelling, if it does occur, is minimal. There may also be sharp pain after strenuous physical activity, such as running or playing a racket sport. If the condition is left untreated for a long period of time, the pain may become much sharper and may be present most of the time, even when the victim is just walking.

Once plantar fasciitis has reached an acute stage, all athletic activity must cease because of the excruciating pain, and the condition may have to be treated more aggressively with anti-inflammatory drugs and/or laser therapy (not laser surgery). Cortisone injections into the heel or surgery are last resorts. Regardless of the aggressive treatments used, they must be accompanied by a solution to the biomechanical fault that caused the problem in the first place. Therefore, people who have developed plantar fasciitis must wear proper footwear and orthotics to prevent the condition from either worsening or recurring. Those involved in any athletic endeavors will have to ensure that their condition has healed before undertaking the activities again.

Recovery time for plantar fasciitis will depend on its severity. If the condition is mild, the patient should be relatively symptom-free within a few weeks, providing proper footwear and orthotics are worn. If the inflammation is more acute and has persisted for a long time, recovery could take up to three months or, in the worst cases, even longer.

In the overwhelming majority of cases, with proper treatment the periosteum (the lining of the bone) will reattach to the bone and the healing will be complete, even though some mild discomfort in the morning may linger. But that too will gradually disappear, and the plantar fasciitis should not recur as long as orthotics and proper footwear are worn.

Out of Joint

Although ankle troubles are more common in sports other than running, a runner can sprain the joint, often severely, by taking a bad step. It can happen on a surface that is not level or that is fairly rough,

and is most frequently due to decreased visibility when one is running at night.

A sprained ankle is actually a sprained ligament. Remember that a ligament is a fibrous band of connective tissue that links bones together at a joint. Ligaments have very little give (although they are somewhat flexible), so they cannot naturally lengthen to accommodate extra pressure placed upon them. If you "turn" your ankle as you are running, you place undue stress on the ligaments of the ankle joint. When this happens, the ligament is either stretched beyond its limits and becomes "sprained" or, in the worst-case scenario, is torn completely away from its moorings.

There are three ligaments in the ankle area that are commonly stretched or torn when the ankle is turned in an inversion sprain. The one most likely to be damaged is the *anterior talo-fibular ligament*. When the injury first occurs, it is often very difficult to properly diagnose whether it is a tear or a sprain, because the swelling and the pain in the area prevent proper manipulation of the joint. The only way to manipulate the area adequately would be to put the patient under a general anesthetic and then play with the ankle. However, such a procedure is rarely, if ever, necessary.

The general philosophy for treatment of a sprained ankle can best be summed up by the acronym RICE (if you are on a protein diet, you will have to cheat). Rest, ice, compression, and elevation are the four main components of the treatment, at least for the first three days after the injury. *Rest* is necessary to give the ankle area a chance to calm down, because any weight on the offending foot will only exacerbate the inflammation. *Ice* is essential to keep down the swelling caused by the inflammation, and it also acts as an analgesic to reduce pain. Icing should be done for fifteen to twenty minutes three or four times a day. *Compression,* by bandaging the injured area, aids in keeping down swelling and internal bleeding caused by the injury. *Elevation* of the foot allows for improved venous and lymphatic flow out of the area. It also reduces swelling in the area and therefore limits loss of motion in the ankle joint.

When one of its ligaments has been damaged, a podiatrist or physical therapist can show you a special way to tape the ankle: the high basket weave. This method of bandaging provides excellent support for the ankle joint and enables the injured person to put weight on the foot much sooner than if a conventional elastic bandage were applied. The bandage should be left on for about a month, although it must be removed and reapplied periodically to allow the area to be examined and to let the skin "breathe."

If proper treatment is begun at the outset of the injury, physiotherapy can be started two to three weeks after the accident, even in cases of moderate to severe ankle-ligament sprains. Laser therapy works well, and it should coincide with stretching exercises to allow the ankle joint to return to full mobility as soon as possible. Most importantly, special exercises are required to return to normal the *proprioceptors* of the ankle. Proprioceptors are sensory nerve endings that monitor internal changes in the body resulting from movement, particularly muscular activity. When the ankle joint is injured, the proprioceptors in the area are damaged and, because the offending foot continues to be unstable, the ankle appears to have been weakened. I wish I had a hundred dollars for every time I have seen patients who were told that their injured ankles were not healing properly because the ligament had not returned to normal. In most cases the ligament has healed properly, but the proprioceptors are still unable to inform the foot where the rest of the leg intends to go. As a result, when the person is walking, the foot does not land where it is supposed to. The results can be painful or comical, depending on whether you are the victim or a not very sympathetic spectator.

Incidentally, I get a lot of questions about ankles from people who run indoors or on small outdoor tracks or paths. If you are constantly turning on a track that has, for example, a dozen or more laps to the mile, are you more prone to overstressing the ankle than if you run on a long, straight pathway or a quarter-mile track? The answer is a qualified yes.

Indoor tracks in particular are often well banked at the corners to conserve energy and cut running times. While you may run farther faster, the banking produces excess pronation in the leg and foot that are higher on the turn than in the other leg and foot. So it is possible to exacerbate an existing biomechanical fault, or even to create one. Such a fault, like overpronation, will eventually result in increased pull on the muscles, tendons, and ligaments in the ankle area and in other parts of the leg and foot.

If you do run indoors, try to avoid severely banked tracks. Also, alternate directions frequently to avoid stressing one leg too much. Doing so may cause traffic jams on the track, but that is better than sore ankles or knees. Of course, if you change directions repeatedly, but still run for a long time on a steeply banked, very hard surface, you may wind up with damage to both lower limbs.

Synovitis of the Ankle Joint

As you know from Chapter 4, synovitis is an inflammation of the outer lining of a joint. Sometimes abnormal pronation can cause the head of the tibia to impinge on the ankle joint, particularly in runners who exaggerate a biomechanical fault as they constantly pound their feet on hard pavement. The result can be ankle-joint synovitis. Ice, ultrasound, and other forms of therapy will not do much good to correct this condition in the long run, because the biomechanical fault must be corrected in order to eliminate the cause of the inflammation. The best way to obtain permanent relief from the synovitis caused by a biomechanical fault is to be fitted with a proper shoe insert.

Tarsal Tunnel Syndrome

We discussed tarsal tunnel syndrome in detail in Chapter 7, in particular how difficult it can be to diagnose. The condition involves impingement of the posterior tibial nerve in the area of the deltoid ligament, on the medial side (inside) of the foot. A runner can develop numbness and tingling sensations in the area of the pinched nerve, as well as along the bottom of the foot and the toes, because abnormal pronation strains the ligament, which then begins to press on the nerve. However, it takes about three to four miles of running before the symptoms appear, so it is extremely difficult to diagnose unless the runner with the problem jogs directly into the doctor's office after a lengthy, painful run.

As I mentioned in Chapter 7, the primary treatment for tarsal tunnel syndrome is wearing correctly fitting running shoes and using orthotics. In rare cases, the nerve can become so inflamed by constant impingement that surgery may be required to widen the tarsal tunnel and/or redirect the nerve through a less congested area.

Because running is so unforgiving of abnormal pronation, the nonrunner can often get away with up to a five-degree pronation without symptoms, whereas a runner will suffer the consequences of even a three-degree pronation. I rarely see tarsal tunnel syndrome in nonathletes. And, fortunately, I see only five or six runners per year with the syndrome.

Achilles Tendonitis

The Achilles tendon attaches at the heel bone (calcaneus) and develops into the gastrocnemius and soleus muscles in the calf. Achilles tendonitis develops for two reasons: The tendon is gradually shortened by constant wearing of high-heeled shoes, or it is shortened when twisted by abnormal pronation. Female athletes who have worn high-heeled shoes almost exclusively for many years may well be cursed with both causes. Athletes who "abuse" their bodies by "overdoing it" will develop Achilles tendonitis from overuse.

I refer the reader to Chapter 7 for a full discussion of the condition. If the primary cause of Achilles tendonitis is abnormal pronation, neither stretching nor physiotherapy will help, because the biomechanical fault will remain. Any treatment program must include a precise evaluation and correction of the abnormal pronation that caused the inflammation. The optimum treatment is to wear proper footwear with prescribed orthotic inserts.

As with other lower-limb conditions, it is vital to treat Achilles tendonitis properly before the inflammation becomes acute. Because of limited blood flow (poor circulation) to that part of the body, the healing process can be quite lengthy and uncomfortable. Such treatments as heel lifts or cushions, anti-inflammatories either injected or taken orally, or surgery to remove "calcium buildup" are ill-advised, since the underlying cause of the problem—abnormal pronation—remains unresolved. When treated properly with prescribed orthotics, Achilles tendonitis should resolve itself within a few weeks. After that, there may be occasional twinges of pain in the area, which can be easily alleviated with ice, but nothing serious enough to curtail sensible athletic activity.

Shin Splints

Like plantar fasciitis, a shin splint is really periostitis (tearing of the lining of the bone away from the bone). It occurs between the knee and ankle joints (see Figure 11.1). As I mentioned earlier, shin splints were extremely common when high-impact aerobic exercising was popular and runners were less educated about the perils of overuse syndromes.

There are two different variations of this condition: medial (tibialis posterior) and lateral (tibialis anterior). The variation depends on where the periosteum is being torn away from the tibia, and by which muscle in the leg.

The tibialis posterior ("tib post") muscle runs down the inside of the leg from the tibia to the bottom of the foot. At the bottom its tendon attaches to the base of the first four metatarsal bones. It is a major antipronating muscle—that is, it helps prevent the lower leg and foot from overpronating. However, when there is abnormal pronation in the rearfoot, the tib post muscle and tendon can become overworked, particularly when the person who overpronates engages in exercise that places undue stress on the legs and feet—for example, running or high-impact aerobics.

When the tib post muscle is overused, it becomes tight. Its tendon is then forced to stretch abnormally to keep it from tearing. Since the attachment of a tendon to its muscle is stronger than its attachment to bone, the tib post tendon begins to pull away from the tibia. The periosteum tears away from the tibia, and the result is painful periostitis: shin splints.

If the shin splints are left untreated and the person continues to overuse the leg, the tib post tendon may eventually rupture, causing complete flattening of the foot; the person will overpronate violently and appear to be walking on the ankle bone. This situation is very difficult to treat and may require surgery to fuse the ankle, which will prevent the foot from overpronating, but will also eliminate the ankle joint's normal range of motion. Therefore the logical approach is to prevent such an injury from occurring in the first place or at least to treat it immediately.

The second type of shin splint is the anterior, or tibialis anterior. As you can see in the diagram, the "tib ant" muscle runs down the outside of the leg and foot from the tibia to the metatarsal bones. It also acts

Figure 11.1. Shin splints

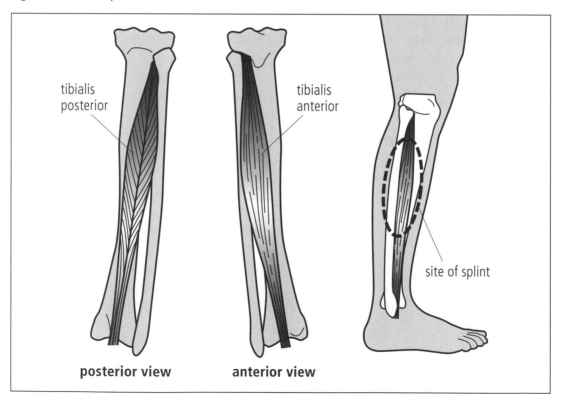

tibialis posterior

tibialis anterior

site of splint

posterior view   **anterior view**

as an antipronation muscle, and it can be adversely affected by abnormal pronation in the foot. However, anterior shin splints are more commonly caused by the muscle itself rather than the foot. Obviously, pain in tib ant periostitis occurs on the outside rather than the inside of the leg.

Correcting abnormal pronation and advising the person how to avoid overuse syndromes can prevent shin splints from occurring, or can at least catch them before they become severe. If, however, the problem has already arisen, the first step in treating a shin splint is to evaluate the person's gait on the computer, and then correct abnormal pronation with a prescribed orthotic. Shin splints may also require further treatment to relieve symptoms of the inflammation; this will usually entail rest, ice, ultrasound, and perhaps even cold laser therapy.

As mentioned above, failure to treat shin splints correctly can lead to a ruptured tendon. It can also result in stress fractures of either the tibia or the fibula. It is important to realize that the "no pain, no gain" notion of exercising is absurd. Pain is nature's way of telling you that something is amiss, not that you need to increase your pain-tolerance level.

Anterior Compartment Syndrome

If you are not an athlete or a medical professional, you may never have heard of anterior compartment syndrome. This condition can be confused with shin splints because, as you can see in Figure 11.2, the anterior compartment (medical-ese for "a part or section in the front") is in the front part of the lower leg.

Since the advent of sports medicine as a discipline of its own, anterior compartment syndrome has come to mean many different things. Now any pain in the area, such as an anterior tibial shin splint, is often diagnosed as an anterior compartment problem. As you can see in Figure 11.2, there are many muscles in the anterior compartment, with different, smaller compartments between them. When any of those muscles inflame and swell, they increase the pressure within the compartments. This increased pressure may cause a mild decrease of blood flow and, therefore, some mild pain. This is what occurs in 99 percent of such cases, and it is rare for surgical intervention to be necessary. An acute anterior compartment syndrome—wherein no blood reaches the compartment because the major artery providing oxygenated blood to the area is pinched off—is a medical emergency. Today, however, the term *anterior compartment syndrome* is often used to describe other disorders, such as shin splints.

If the condition is mild, the discomfort and inflammation can be alleviated with rest, ice, and easy stretching of the leg. But it can recur unless the cause of the problem is addressed. The most common causes are poor biomechanics of the lower limbs; ill-fitting shoes; ineffective or insufficient warm-up, stretching, and cool-down

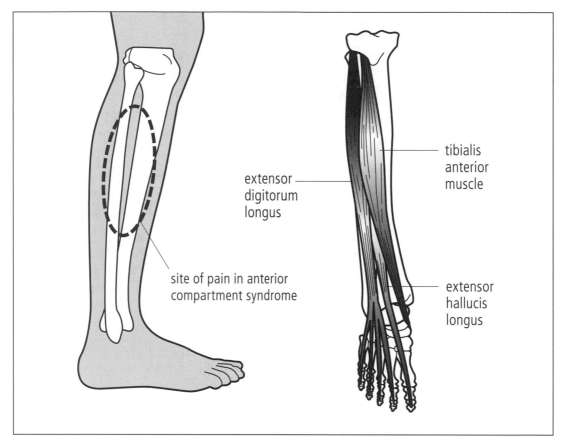

Figure 11.2. Anterior compartment syndrome

exercises; and overuse. I advise all runners, and indeed all serious athletes, to pay attention to the need for proper stretching before and after engaging in strenuous activity. This will help you avoid anterior compartment syndrome, particularly if you have a biomechanical disorder.

If the anterior compartment syndrome persists despite all the treatment and preventive measures, in the most serious, chronic cases it may be necessary to operate to decompress the compartment—that is, to enlarge the space through which the

impinged blood vessel must pass. However, this is a rare occurrence; there is no need to worry unduly if you suffer from the syndrome but have not yet taken all the steps necessary to control it.

The Chondromalacia Generation: Runner's Knee

The most common term for chondromalacia patella is "runner's knee," because it is so closely associated with the running and jogging craze that began three decades ago.

Chondromalacia patella is caused by faulty biomechanics of the legs and foot. In the case of runners, abnormal pronation forces the patellar tendon to be pulled to the inside by internal rotation of the lower leg. At the same time, the upper part of the leg is rotating externally—which is normal—and it is unable to compensate for the abnormal pronation of the lower leg. Thus the upper part of the leg is twisting the knee joint to the outside, while the lower part of the leg is twisting it to the inside. As you can see in Figure 11.3, the patella (kneecap) normally moves up and down within a groove that lies between both the medial and lateral femoral condyles, which are rounded protuberances at the end of the femur bone. The external rotation of the femur with the simultaneous internal rotation of the patellar tendon yanks the patella out of its normal track between the condyles. When this occurs, the patella begins rubbing on the condyles, and the cartilage on the back of the patella is subjected to severely abnormal wear and tear.

The most common symptoms of chondromalacia patella are:

● acute pain radiating from the top of the kneecap, particularly when walking up or down stairs;

● stiffness in the knee joint after two or more hours of sitting with a bent leg and then bearing weight on that leg;

● reduced mobility of the knee joint so that the normal range of motions is restricted.

Treatment for chondromalacia patella, regardless of its severity, should include orthotics to eliminate abnormal pronation. Because of its dynamic measurement of the patient's gait—the biomechanics of the foot and leg—the computerized technique is the obvious choice for accurate diagnosis and treatment of the condition. It may be necessary to combine orthotic treatment with therapies to relieve inflammation and build up muscles in the leg. Surgery is necessary only if the condition has progressed to the point where the knee joint has become irreparably damaged because the cartilage has almost completely worn out and bone is grinding against bone.

As with other conditions that can be either caused or exacerbated by "overuse," it is important for the runner or other athlete not to continue his or her activity while in pain. Doing that will only cause further deterioration in the knee joint, which may result in either a much longer recovery time or subsequent inability to partake in a favorite physical activity.

Although runner's knee will not necessarily show up on X rays, particularly early ones, the condition has some obvious symptoms, as we noted above. Treatment will depend on the primary causes of the problem, which often act together to promote dysfunction of the knee joint: weak or malfunctioning quadriceps muscles above the knee, faulty biomechanics of the foot and lower leg, and a dysfunctional patellar tendon below the knee. I will concentrate on the biomechanical problems.

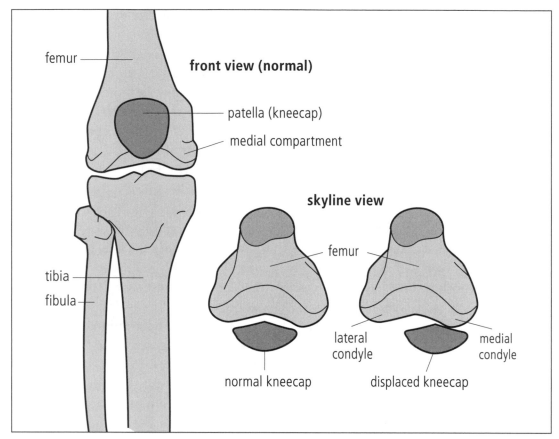

Figure 11.3. The kneecap and the medial compartment

A foot that pronates abnormally tends to turn the knee to the inside. When this happens, there is undue stress on the knee joint itself. As the leg tries to compensate for the abnormal pronation, the kneecap may deviate from its normal path in its groove. Another factor in the development of runner's knee may be poor alignment of the patellar tendon with the knee joint. This may also be caused by abnormal pronation, which forces the tendon out of alignment as it attempts to compensate for the biomechanical fault.

There are a few less common causes of runner's knee. The runner may be wearing ill-fitting shoes that by themselves induce a biomechanical fault, or running on banked or uneven rough surfaces that can accentuate a biomechanical fault and cause pulling on the knee joint. Running up or down hills will also add to stress on the knee, which must be bent constantly to adjust to the sloping terrain. It has been determined scientifically that the forces on the leg multiply threefold when a person runs uphill, and fivefold for downhill. It is easy to understand why runners and other serious athletes are far more prone to foot and leg problems than nonexercisers.

When I see a case of runner's knee, the first thing I must do after making the diagnosis is find the cause. Once I have determined the cause of the complaint, I can advise the patient as to the proper corrective measures and therapy to take. If the cause is a biomechanical fault, orthotics in the running shoes are indicated, and the runner must be advised of the proper shoes to wear (I discuss athletic shoes in detail in Chapter 15).

Many people with runner's knee have found relief with various braces, straps, and other paraphernalia to keep the knee joint in proper alignment. These appliances may indeed help relieve mild pain, but they do not correct the underlying causes of the disorder. I strongly recommend that you seek expert medical advice before relying solely on such aids to treat runner's knee or any other knee condition.

Tibial Pursuit

Runners who are slightly bowlegged (tibial varum) or knock-kneed (tibial valgum) are prone to problems they would not be subject to under normal walking conditions. This is, of course, because of the extra stress placed on the legs while running, particularly on hilly or uneven terrain.

One of these problems is osteoarthritis of the knee. If the runner is bowlegged, all of the body weight may be transferred to the medial (inside) compartment of the knee, because the position of the feet is inverted to compensate for the shape of the leg. If the problem is one of knock knees, the runner may overpronate and force the body weight onto the lateral (outside) compartment of the knee. When either of these conditions occur, the overstressed side of the knee joint wears down while the other side remains as good as new. Osteoarthritis in the knee joint will probably produce profound discomfort in the area of inflammation. X rays of the knee joint should confirm the presence of the condition.

The treatment for this problem is to reduce the inflammation with physiotherapy and/or oral anti-inflammatory drugs. At the same time, the biomechanical fault of the lower limbs must be dealt with. Orthotic devices will compensate for overpronation or abnormal supination and will help keep the legs as straight as possible. It is important to exercise and stretch the quadriceps muscles and the hamstrings, as they also help keep the leg properly aligned. If permanent wear and tear has occurred, modern surgery techniques may be able to repair much of the damage. Again, it is important for athletes to remember that if they are experiencing pain in the knee area during exercise, they should seek medical advice as soon as possible to determine the cause of the problem, and to avoid a potentially lasting disorder in the knee joint.

And the Band Frayed On

The *iliotibial band* is a stretch of muscular tissue that runs from the hip joint down the outside of the leg and attaches into the head of the fibula, just below the knee. One function of this band is to prevent internal rotation of the leg and thigh, and it is vital for runners, because they place heavy, repetitive stress on their legs with every stride.

If the iliotibial band, which runs over the outside part of the knee joint, is stretched too tightly, it will become irritated by the friction that occurs when it contacts the kneecap. If it is poorly developed or very short, the band may be overstretched because it is abnormally tight to begin with. A badly overpronating foot will produce an internally rotating leg, and this situation will also unduly stress the band. Occasionally iliotibial-band friction syndrome is caused by too much running up and down hills or by constant running on uneven, rough terrain.

The symptoms of the syndrome are pain and tenderness on the outside of the knee, at the head of the fibula and upwards. The symptoms may approximate runner's knee, because walking up and down stairs produces pain and there is stiffness in the knee joint after sitting with knees bent for more than a couple of hours. However, the pain will be located more on the outside of the joint. Some medical experts believe that the discomfort is caused by an inflammation of the bursa, the small sac of fibrous tissue filled with synovial fluid that is situated where friction is caused by ligaments or tendons that pass over bones. This particular bursa lies between the iliotibial band and the lateral side of the knee joint.

The treatment for iliotibial-band friction syndrome is a program of exercises to properly stretch the band; ice and ultrasound to relieve the discomfort; a change in footwear, possibly including orthotics to correct a biomechanical fault; and a change in running habits to avoid the more stressful conditions.

A Pain in the Butt

The sciatic nerve exits from the spinal column and runs down the leg. In the disorder known as *sciatica,* this nerve is pinched either in the low back or somewhere in its path down the leg. The syndrome produces aches, pains, and occasional numb, tingling sensations down the leg and into the toes.

Until a few years ago it was thought that all cases of sciatica originated from impingement of the sciatic nerve in the lower back by a protruding disc or a facet joint abnormality in the spinal column. But it is now generally accepted that nerve impingement can also take place in the upper part of the leg, specifically where the nerve runs under the piriformis muscle (see Figure 11.4). This muscle acts to prevent the femur (thigh bone) from rotating internally, a problem that occurs in runners with biomechanical faults in their lower limbs. When the femur over-rotates, excess stress is placed on the piriformis muscle, which then tightens and binds down on the sciatic nerve. The nerve becomes irritated, and pain from the inflammation radiates from the source of the problem—in the area of the buttocks—and can travel down the leg, behind the knee, and into the foot. This is known as *piriformis syndrome.*

In my clinical experience with piriformis syndrome, when I am able to correct the internal rotation of the femur with orthotics, I have a high success rate in controlling the sciatic pain. Naturally, this course of action is taken only after an exhaustive examination of the patient has ruled out a lower-back problem. I also advise the runner to undertake a proper exercise program, stretching the piriformis muscle to help prevent it from impinging on the sciatic nerve. A good athletic therapist can provide you with the proper set of exercises.

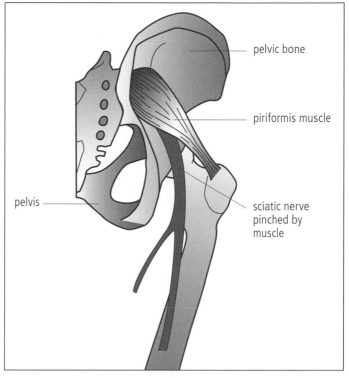

Figure 11.4. Piriformis syndrome

More clinical studies are being published that lend credence to the theory that piriformis syndrome causes sciatic pain. I suspect that, as with runner's knee, we will be hearing a lot more about this condition in the next few years. It is certainly becoming more common as running again becomes popular.

Chapter 12

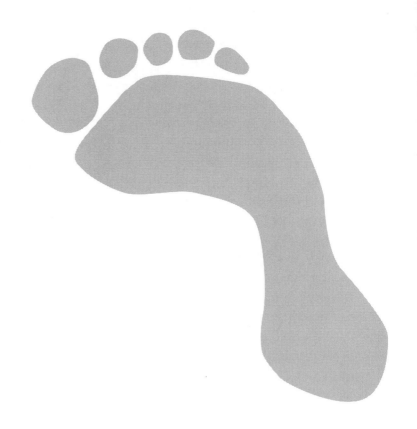

Athletes' Feet II:
Other Sports

I would guess that the majority of readers interested in this subject will want to turn directly to the physical activity in which they engage. To that end, I have divided the chapter into categories of physical activities. However, I advise you to read about all the athletic activities discussed here, as someday you may no longer be able to carry on your favorite sport, or you may be considering a new exercise program for the first time.

Aerobics

It is time to turn our attention to aerobics. Many condition-conscious people have decided against running as a way of developing their bodies, and have turned instead to aerobic exercising in one form or another: high-impact, low-impact, step; treadmills, stair-climbers, elliptical machines, and a whole host of other contraptions designed to get you into shape.

Too many unfit people join clubs and immediately jump into aerobics classes and other exercise regimens, totally unprepared for the strain that the exercises subject their bodies to. And, alas, too many aerobics teachers on the circuit still do not know how to conduct a class properly and are unwilling or ill-prepared to tailor their classes to the needs of the individual participants.

Some people do their aerobic exercises at home, to the often impossible urgings of an instructor on videotape or television. There are two major problems with this type of exercising. First, there is no trainer present to tell you if you are doing something wrong, and you are therefore more prone to injury. Second, many people try to do too much too soon, trying to keep up with the tapes or with the unbelievably fit instructors on the television screen.

I am not against aerobic exercising. I only caution you to do the exercises correctly, and in accordance with your physical condition. Aerobics is a marvelous way of getting into shape and helping you shed unwanted weight without having to go on a starvation diet. Moreover, by increasing your cardiovascular and pulmonary capacities with the vigorous exercise aerobic activities provide, you stand a good chance of feeling better both mentally and physically, and therefore you are better able to cope with the anxieties of life in the fast lane. And—who knows?—you may even meet the love of your life in one of those sweaty exercise classes.

Because of the tremendous amount of stress to the lower extremities from constantly repeating the same movements, a common concern for those who do aerobics is shin splints. We have discussed how the periosteum—the tough outer layer, or lining, of soft tissue that covers the tibia (the shinbone)—is torn away from the bone by the abnormal pulling force of either the tibialis posterior or the tibialis anterior muscle, where its tendon attaches to the tibia. We have also discussed how abnormal pronation, in particular, puts extra stress on the involved tendon as it tries to keep the leg straight during any

Chapter 12: Athletes' Feet II—Other Sports

form of exercise that involves constant pounding on the feet.

In many types of aerobic exercising the feet absorb a tremendous number of repeated shocks. Therefore, there is an excellent possibility that shin splints will develop. Fortunately, high-impact aerobics seem to be largely going the way of the dodo—replaced by low-impact or step aerobics—which means that the incidence of shin splints has dropped dramatically in the past couple of years. So people who do aerobics need not develop shin splints on a regular basis. All they have to do is take the proper precautions.

First of all—and this applies to all athletes, all of the time—do not try to do too much too soon! Most aerobics injuries are caused by "overuse" syndrome: overexercising parts of the body that are ill-prepared for the stress. So if you are a beginner and you have joined a club that has no introductory classes, ask for your money back quickly and seek out another club that will provide classes tailored to your needs.

It is equally important, even in beginners' classes, that the instructor knows how to conduct proper warm-ups and stretching so that your body is prepared for the more difficult routines that follow. As far as the lower extremities are concerned, it is vital to stretch the tibialis anterior and posterior muscles and the Achilles tendon before you begin bouncing around the floor, or you could end up with Achilles tendonitis or a related problem.

Even if you do not have a biomechanical foot problem, it is essential to use the proper footwear when doing aerobic exercises. Otherwise you will lack the stability to prevent your feet from rolling too much during the routines. Remember, biomechanical faults that do not cause trouble when you are merely walking can suddenly cause all sorts of problems when your feet are subjected to additional stresses and are forced to absorb much more shock than normal.

Another common problem for people doing aerobics is Achilles tendonitis, often because the tendon is not properly stretched before the class gets into the difficult routines. And again, there is the problem of overuse and doing too much too soon. Women, in particular, are prone to this complaint because many of them have worn predominantly high-heeled shoes for years, then have suddenly decided to take up aerobic exercising to get their bodies back in shape. They are trying to do the exercises on Achilles tendons that have shrunk from misuse during their years on the high heels. So they develop inflamed tendons and are forced to give up exercising altogether until the tendonitis clears up, weeks later. By that time they have probably, and sadly, given up exercising for good. And all because they did too much, too soon on Achilles tendons that were not properly stretched before they were subjected to undue stress from the exercises.

You will recall that stress fractures of the tibia and the fibula can occur when the

148 The Good Foot Book

tendons attached to them become so inflamed that they exert tremendous force on the bones. When this force becomes overwhelming, the bone gives, and stress fractures occur. The two major tendons involved in these types of fractures are those of the tibialis posterior and tibialis anterior muscles (see Figure 11.1, page 138). These fractures can take up to a year to heal. One of the problems involved with recovery is misdiagnosis of the fractures, because they do not always show up on X rays. The patient is often treated first for shin splints, because the pain is in the same area. However, the telltale sign of a fracture is that application of ultrasound (to treat the supposed shin splints) will enhance the pain, rather than relieve it. It may then be necessary to do a bone scan to isolate the break, although after a few weeks it ought to show up on regular X rays.

The best treatment for stress fractures of the tibia, the fibula, or the metatarsals is prevention. Do not try to exercise through pain, because pain is nature's way of telling you that something is amiss in your body. None of these fractures will have to be put in a cast, so you will not suffer aesthetically, but the discomfort from the fractures can be quite acute, and can last for a few months.

Racket Sports

The damage done to the lower limbs of racket-sports players ranks right up there with that caused by running and aerobics.

The major reasons for racket-sports injuries to the legs and feet are the dramatic stop-and-start movements required to chase the balls, the hard surfaces on which the games are played, and the players' lack of proper conditioning. As well, in tennis there is an increased risk of sesamoiditis because of the great amount of pressure on the area of the first metatarsal head while serving. Professional tennis players, who often serve over a hundred times per match, are generally quite prone to inflamed sesamoids, because these bones lie right under the first metatarsal head. The next time you watch a tennis match, observe how the biomechanics of the tennis serve stress this area of the foot.

Because of all the lateral stop-and-go movements made by racket-sports players, "inversion" ankle sprains are not uncommon. The same lateral movements place an extra load on the Achilles tendon, which is already working hard to prevent ankle instability, and can cause Achilles tendonitis. The dramatic stopping and starting, combined with hard running on unyielding surfaces, can cause plantar fasciitis—the player is constantly "planting" the heel of the foot for stability and leverage when making a shot.

In the forefoot, racket-sports players are prone to toenail problems, because the sudden stops cause the ends of the toes to slam into the front of the shoe. Aside from the toenails, the bottoms of the forefeet are subjected to tremendous pressure as the player slides laterally from side to side, creating friction between the foot, the shoe, and the court surface. It is thus not uncommon to see competitive players with feet full of calluses and blisters. And, because of the extra stress on the forefoot, racket-sports players are also more likely than others to suffer from forefoot neuromas. The entire forefoot is constantly being impinged by the rapid, jerky movements required in a fast-moving match, and the nerves in the forefoot are fair game for irritation caused by the suddenly cramped spaces through which they must pass.

Finally, the entire lower part of the body of a racket-sports player is subjected to extra pounding by constant running and stop-and-start actions on hard surfaces. Any biomechanical fault that might otherwise not bother a person will probably create havoc in a racket-sports athlete. I have treated one tennis player continually for years for various foot and leg problems. He tells me that he can play all day on clay surfaces because they are yielding, and therefore less demanding in terms of shock absorption. However, he can play only a few minutes on an asphalt court before he starts to experience all sorts of aches and pains, all the way up to his lower back. Unfortunately, very few matches these days are played on clay surfaces.

Dance

Although ballet dancers may not be classified as athletes, they are certainly as well conditioned and aware of their bodies as any sports enthusiast. I have treated a number of ballet dancers for various foot problems over the years, and they are definitely in better shape than many of the athletes I see in my practice. Ballet dancers often have foot and leg problems (and some of the ugliest feet), although generally these are cumulative injuries, developed during years of continuous straining of the lower limbs to perform movements for which the body was not designed. They also often have overdeveloped muscles, required to prevent instability in the feet while dancing.

The most common problem in female dancers is hammer toes. Because there is a tremendous amount of pressure on the toes in dancing on pointe, the flexor and extensor muscles of the toes become overdeveloped and tight. When this happens, all the digits contract, forming hammer toes. Of course, the only way to really prevent this is to stop dancing on pointed toes. But then what would become of ballet dancing?

As you might expect, another common complaint of ballet dancers is osteoarthritis of the toe joints because of the tremendous stress to those joints during dancing. It is almost inevitable that ballet dancers will suffer early wear and tear of the toe joints.

The third major condition affecting female ballet dancers is traumatized toenails. If you spent a good part of your workday on your toes, you would also suffer from toenail abnormalities. Ballet dancers are plagued by all three of the most common toenail problems: ingrown, mycotic (fungal), and gryphotic (misshapen) nails. These conditions are the badges of honor for ballet dancers—the price they have to pay for the rewards of their profession.

Ballet dancers also tend to develop soft corns between their toes. The toes are constantly being squeezed together, and friction between the toes will cause corn growth to protect the irritated skin.

Because ballet dancers are generally in excellent condition and know how to warm up and stretch properly, they usually avoid missteps and twisted ankles. However, they can suffer from various types of tendonitis, strictly from overuse of their lower limbs during exhausting training and/or performances.

Aside from ballet, other types of dancing can be just as hard on the lower extremities. Other dancers are rarely as fit as ballet dancers, but they often try moves for which their bodies were neither designed nor prepared. Certain forms of modern dance as well as aerobic exercises such as dancercise are very hard on the lower limbs. It is not uncommon to see these other dancers with severe cases of plantar fasciitis and shin splints because they have not warmed up properly before doing strenuous dance moves.

Basketball and Volleyball

I have lumped basketball and volleyball together because most of the associated complaints seem to be similar in nature and are caused by the same types of problems. Basketball and volleyball players tend to be prone to plantar fasciitis and Achilles tendonitis because they do not properly stretch their lower limbs before beginning to play. There is a lot of jumping and stop-and-start movement associated with these sports. The lower limbs will be subjected to much undue stress if the stability of the ankles and feet is undermined by underdeveloped muscles and tendons around the ankle. Coincidentally, these athletes often suffer from sprained ankles because of inverted landings after jumping for a ball, even though the high-topped shoes they now wear do provide more stability in the area.

Besides wearing proper shoes, the remedy for these conditions is an exercise program designed to develop the muscles and tendons around the ankle to provide the required stability in the area. If you have had an ankle injury, you will also want to do the exercises for the proprioceptors that I mentioned on page 135. A physiotherapist can develop an exercise program for your specific needs.

Basketball and volleyball players tend to be more susceptible than other athletes to capsulitis under the metatarsal heads. This is probably caused by the added stress placed on the forefoot as the player prepares to jump for a ball. If there is a biomechanical fault in the forefoot, it will be exaggerated by this preparatory setting of the feet, and it should be treated with a proper shoe insert.

Football

Most of the foot injuries in football are traumatic. Players get stomped on, accidentally or otherwise, or they twist an ankle on unyielding turf. It is amazing, considering the mayhem that occurs during a football game, that the players do not suffer more severe, debilitating injuries. One of the reasons may be that football players have exceedingly strong thighs and lower legs, and these well-developed muscles help prevent joint and muscle/tendon injuries. Strong muscles help keep the joints in their proper alignment; properly stretched muscles help prevent tendonitis.

Another problem that football players—and other athletes playing on artificial turf—have to contend with is "turf toe." This is not a dermatological problem, and the affected toe does not take on a grassy appearance. It is a condition brought on by the unyielding quality of artificial surfaces that have been laid down on a field, supposedly to provide better traction in inclement weather, and to reduce overall maintenance costs.

Unfortunately, artificial turf has very little give. When an athlete plants a foot in order to change direction or obtain leverage, it tends to stay planted. When this happens, the big-toe joint can get jammed and an irritation of the cartilage can develop. This irritation can develop into synovitis or capsulitis, particularly if the athlete repeatedly jams a toe while trying to "make a cut"—to quickly change direction by planting one foot firmly in the turf. In the good old days of sports fields made of real grass, when an athlete made a cut, there was enough give in the turf to prevent his toe from jamming when he pushed off the foot. If the ground was wet and slippery, he would lose his grip on the turf and slip or fall down. But there would be no undue pressure on the big-toe joint.

Treatment for turf toe is difficult as long as the athlete keeps playing on artificial turf. However, certain steps can be taken. First, it has been clinically proven that the athletes most likely to suffer from turf toe have what are called plantar-flexed first metatarsals, the biomechanical fault in which the first metatarsal stays down at all times instead of moving in unison with the other metatarsals. This causes there to be more weight on the first metatarsal head than there ought to be, and the area receives greater stress than normal. This means there is an increased chance of inflammation occurring, particularly when the area is traumatized. It would be prudent for an athlete with such a condition to have it treated with an orthotic device, particularly when he or she is playing fairly frequently on artificial turf. It would also be wise for the player prone to turf toe to wear shoes with shorter cleats, so that they will give way rather than dig deep into the turf and cause the big toe to jam more.

If the condition requires therapy, ice and ultrasound will often help relieve the inflammation. If the condition is severe, it may be necessary to treat it with an oral anti-inflammatory drug. Turf toe, if left untreated, can lead to hallux limitus or hallux rigidus. Once this happens, the player may eventually require surgery to alleviate the discomfort.

Artificial turf also contributes to increased injuries of other joints such as the ankle and knee, when players' spikes catch in the unyielding surface and soft tissues such as muscles, tendons, and ligaments are stretched or twisted beyond capacity. Thanks to artificial surfaces, torn Achilles tendons, which used to be rare in sports, are on the increase.

Gymnastics

Gymnasts are usually in excellent condition—when they are fully mature physically. The problem is that too many youngsters in serious gymnastic training are trying to do too much before their bodies have developed properly. They are overstressing muscles and tendons that have not kept up with bone growth. Muscles and tendons that are too short to securely attach to fully developed skeletal forms become overstressed and inflamed. So, as a result of overuse of underdeveloped bodies, it is not uncommon to see repeated cases of Achilles tendonitis, plantar fasciitis, and ankle sprains in these youngsters. Prevention here is worth a few pounds of cure. It is important for still-growing youngsters to get the proper coaching so that they are not being forced to overextend themselves.

Another problem for gymnasts, young or otherwise, is metatarsal-head capsulitis. Certain positions on the balance beam or during floor routines and jumping maneuvers place extreme pressure on the forefoot. As with all other strenuous physical activities, problems of poor biomechanics are multiplied exponentially, compared with normal walking. So it is logical for any gymnast with a foot problem to find out whether a biomechanical fault exists, and to treat it accordingly, at once.

Skating

Hockey players are somewhat like football players: They tend to have extremely strong, flexible lower-limb muscles and tendons as a result of strenuous exercising. Therefore, it is not often that I see a hockey player with an injury similar to those incurred by runners and aerobic exercisers. Most foot injuries to hockey players are traumatic, from getting slashed by an "errant" stick or hit by a puck traveling at the speed of sound. On rare occasions they may be gashed by another player's skate.

The players that I see usually have a pronation problem. Although little research has been done on the biomechanics of skating, I have noticed that skaters who overpronate tend to skate with their legs wider apart to compensate for poorer-than-normal balance. Because of this technique, they cannot easily turn quickly or sharply, and their overall ability to compete suffers. I have seen dramatic improvement in the skating abilities of some hockey players after they have been prescribed orthotic devices for their skates. They may not suddenly become Wayne Gretzky, but their newfound mobility on ice may save them some long bus trips to minor-league towns.

Figure skaters are similar to hockey players in that most of the injuries they are likely to suffer are of a traumatic nature. However, I have treated a few world-class figure skaters in Canada who suffered from forefoot neuromas because their skates either were too tight to begin with or were laced up too tightly. Because their skates were so tight, these skaters placed even greater pressure on their forefeet during spins and similar moves that place extra stress on the balls of the feet. The obvious solution to the problem is to wear properly fitting skates and to avoid lacing them up too tightly.

Skiing

By now you should not be surprised to learn that most serious downhill skiers who compete in slalom or downhill events wear orthotics in their ski boots. According to one study I have seen, the figure is about 85 percent. This cannot be too far from accurate, since at least half a dozen major manufacturers of ski equipment make special orthotic devices for ski boots.

The reason for downhill skiers to wear orthotics is that in a normal run down the slopes they are constantly pronating three or four degrees on one foot while simultaneously supinating the same amount on the other foot. The biomechanics of downhill skiing are such that this phenomenon cannot be avoided. A skier would have to have perfectly balanced feet—with absolutely no abnormal pronation or supination—to be able to tolerate the simultaneous extra pronating and supinating of the opposite feet without developing a serious lower-limb problem. So it is natural that most of them require orthotics when skiing. If you have a definite biomechanical foot fault and do a lot of downhill skiing, you would be wise to purchase a pair of special ski-boot orthotics to help protect yourself from potential overstress conditions that may eventually affect your lower limbs.

Many ski shops sell ski-boot orthotics, and I have been in many where the sales personnel knew a lot about the wide range of orthotic devices they carried and why they were required. But I have also been in a few ski shops where the personnel knew absolutely nothing about the biomechanics of skiing. Therefore, make absolutely sure that the ski-equipment store you are dealing with has well-informed salespeople.

Aside from the biomechanical problems inherent in downhill skiing, forefoot neuromas may develop from ski boots that are too tight. As with any footwear, if the boot does not feel comfortable, get into a size and style of boot that keeps your foot stable but does not pinch anywhere. I can never understand why some people are so eager to squeeze into the tightest possible pair of shoes or boots they can find. They are only looking for trouble.

Almost all the other downhill skiing injuries are traumatic, the result of attempting too difficult a slope, using a faulty piece of equipment that causes loss of balance, or just plain bad luck, such as running into a tree that refuses to get out of your way.

Cross-country skiers rarely have injuries that can be related directly to overuse or biomechanical problems. This may be because these athletes are more like ballet dancers and martial arts athletes, who know how to take good care of their bodies. Also, soft snow is much more forgiving than rigid, hard surfaces; a misstep is less likely to lead to a disastrous accident that could affect the lower limbs to any great degree.

Soccer

Soccer is probably the one truly universal game. Almost every country on earth enters a team in the qualifying rounds leading up to the World Cup championships. And, although the sport continuously flops professionally in North America, it is being played more and more by youngsters as a substitute for the costlier—and more injury-producing—game of American football.

Soccer players can develop an interesting list of foot injuries aside from the usual plantar fasciitis, ankle sprain, Achilles tendonitis, and similar overuse syndromes.

But soccer players have fewer overuse injuries than players of most other sports, because they tend to be among the best-conditioned athletes in competitive sports. They have to be able to stand the pace of ninety minutes of constant motion up and down the field. However, they are prone to some injuries caused by the nature of the game, which requires sharp turns, quick stops and starts, kicking the ball from awkward angles, and tackling opponents. The condition of the playing surface is often a factor in soccer injuries to the foot. Rough, hard, uneven surfaces may result in a player taking a misstep, twisting an ankle, and possibly severely damaging an Achilles tendon or a ligament in the process. In North America, many games are played on artificial turf, and soccer players are just as susceptible to turf toe and related injuries as other athletes playing on such surfaces.

When the foot is bent awkwardly back due to a missed kick in which the foot accidentally jams into the ground before the ball, soccer players can suffer from severe tendonitis of the tibialis anterior muscle. They may also be plagued by lateral shin splints because they make more use of the outside of their feet, particularly when "dribbling" the ball as they move forward or laterally. As well, they may develop tendonitis on the peroneus longus and brevis, muscles that lie on the outside lateral part of the leg. These muscles act to prevent inversion of the ankles, and are strained when a player kicks the ball sideways. The way to help prevent these inflammations from occurring is to ensure that the muscles and tendons are properly stretched before the game.

It is also possible for serious soccer players to lose feeling in their toes, usually because their shoes are far too tight. The cramping severely compresses the dorsalis pedis nerve. Unfortunately, this disorder can become permanent if the tight shoes are worn for too long.

Baseball

Since I am consulting podiatrist to the Toronto Blue Jays baseball team, as well as a consultant for many other teams and all the major-league umpires, you might have thought that I would dwell on baseball for pages. However, injuries to the lower extremities are not usually a major concern for most ballplayers, although a few have been plagued by—or had their careers ended by—various foot injuries.

One of the most famous (and eccentric) players of all time, Dizzy Dean, was forced to quit after the big toe on one of his feet was broken by a line drive off the bat of the player to whom he was pitching. He apparently tried to return to action before the toe healed properly, altering his pitching biomechanics to avoid the pain in his foot caused by his old, natural delivery. As a result he threw out his arm, and his career ended abruptly, long before it should have.

Baseball players today are in much better shape than they were a generation ago.

This is because they now spend much more time warming up and stretching before a game. Most of them also engage in specific off-season exercise regimens to keep themselves in good condition for the coming season. However, the game also developed negatively as far as a player's lower limbs are concerned. The culprit is the artificial surface installed on so many stadium floors. Major-league ballplayers now play up to 162 games a year, often going for days without a break. For teams that play on artificial turf at home, the toll on the players' legs is amazing. Because the artificial turf is so unyielding, even the best-conditioned baseball players may eventually succumb to overuse syndromes, such as plantar fasciitis, chondromalacia of the patella, and, to a lesser extent, Achilles tendonitis. Fortunately, most major-league teams, and almost all the minor-league teams, have reverted to natural grass fields, which are much easier on the lower limbs.

As with football, one of the primary scourges of baseball players playing on artificial surfaces is turf toe. They are constantly jamming their big toes into their shoes as they try to change directions sharply and quickly on the artificial turf. Amateur baseball players, and professionals who are lucky enough to play most, if not all, of their games on natural grass, have a very low incidence of foot problems. Because the health of their feet is important to their success as ballplayers, they tend to take good care of them and seek relief for nagging hurts, which generally turn out to be caused by biomechanical problems. A large number of baseball players wear orthotics to correct such problems.

Cycling

Even cyclists can develop lower-limb problems as a result of foot, lower-leg, and knee misalignments. Many of their problems are a result of improper seat height, which can produce dramatically abnormal biomechanics and unpleasant foot, leg, hip, and back discomfort. The simple solution is to adjust the height of the seat or to buy a bicycle that fits you better. If a cyclist has a specific biomechanical abnormality that is exacerbated by riding a bike, orthotics to realign the foot and knee should eliminate the problem.

In-Line Skating

If you have taken up in-line skating—or have almost been bowled over by a skater while out walking—you will know how popular it has become. It is not uncommon these days to see even white-collar workers wheeling their way along busy downtown streets on their way to or from their office.

The problems of in-line skaters often resemble those of skiers because of a similarity in footwear and certain movements. Many in-line skaters believe they have weak ankles, but they are probably overpronators who require orthotics to correct lower-limb abnormalities that affect the ankle and adjacent areas. If they overpronate badly, they may develop pain on the inside of the ankle bone. In-line skate boots can also produce blisters in the arch area if they do not fit properly.

Hiking

Hiking, or trekking, is one of the reinvented activities of the new century. Actually, orienteering races, which combine hiking with long-distance running, have been held for many years in various countries. The sport probably traces its history back to Sweden, from which the word *orienteering* comes. Popular hiking, however, entails walking long distances, often over very uneven terrain. Too many people attempt to hike with improper equipment, particularly their footwear.

Hikers must understand their footwear needs. First and foremost is stability, which is why a high-top boot that fits snugly around the ankle is so important. Because you are navigating on such uneven surfaces, the ankle must remain as stable as possible. Even if you take a bad step and your ankle twists, the boot will be there to stabilize the joint. Just as in basketball and football, where missteps are also common, if you are attempting to hike on very rough terrain, it would be wise to tape your ankles to prevent a sprain or other injury.

One of the unique requirements of hiking boots is the ability of the sole to grip onto surfaces such as wet tree roots and other slippery, uneven surfaces. If you try to hike in running shoes or other athletic footwear, you will probably slip and slide a lot, setting yourself up for nasty fall.

Finally, many hiking boots are touted to be waterproof, which is important if you are on the trails in inclement weather. But while the footwear may keep your lower extremities dry, it is important that the boots also allow your feet to breathe properly. Some waterproof boots hardly allow the feet to breathe at all. The subsequent buildup of perspiration inside the boot creates a haven for fungal growth or other skin inflammations.

A Pitch for Prevention

When it comes to performing the activity of your choice, there are two things to keep in mind. First, establish your goals—long-term and short-term—so that you can accomplish what you have set out to do in a realistic manner. It would be wise to seek expert advice, perhaps from a coach or an instructor, so that you do not bite off more than you can chew.

A trainer is also important to help you avoid athletic injuries. Improper training methods, not traumatic episodes, are the primary causes of sports injuries. A good coach will be able to provide you with proper warm-up and stretching exercises, and teach you what to do to cool down and keep your muscles and tendons stretched after you have finished for the day. A coach will also refine your technique in whatever activity you pursue, so that you will be able to maximize your energy resources while at the same time minimizing the risk of overuse and wear-and-tear syndromes. I have refrained from including specific exercises in this book because I would rather the athlete be shown the exercises by an expert, so that they are done properly.

Finally, there is an old expression, "Enough is as good as a feast." That applies to physical activity as well as to food. One of the most common causes of sports injuries is overuse syndrome.

If you do injure yourself, by either overuse or trauma, remember that it is not wise to exercise through the pain. You will only aggravate the condition and keep yourself out of action for much longer than if you had taken proper precautions at the onset of discomfort. Pain tells you that something is wrong. It is not to test your character—unless, perhaps, you are trying to win the Tour de France.

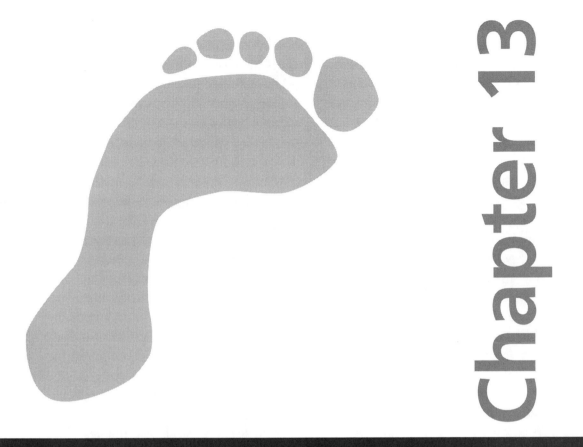

Chapter 13

Dermatological Foot Problems

Chapter 13: Dermatological Foot Problems

The study of skin diseases—dermatology—is a very difficult science. One of the problems in treating these conditions is identifying the correct option from the thousands that exist. Also, these disorders come in a multitude of varieties and erupt on just about any part of the body. Skin diseases (other than cancers) are rarely fatal, so medical research is not generally directed toward finding miracle cures for conditions that may well eventually go away by themselves or respond to treatments that already exist.

Fortunately, most skin disorders of the foot are quite easy to identify and can usually be dealt with by using state-of-the-art treatments. In previous chapters I have discussed certain conditions that could be considered dermatological; these include corns, calluses, and warts. I readily agree that plantar warts are dermatological disorders, but I decided to include them with other conditions affecting the bottom of the foot, because they are often confused with calluses. So what does that leave for this chapter? Well, as you might imagine, there is at least one skin disorder that attacks the foot almost exclusively, and that is *tinea pedis*. Translated from medical Latin, tinea pedis means "a fungus of the foot," but we know it most commonly as athlete's foot.

Athlete's Foot

How did tinea pedis become known as athlete's foot? I suspect it had something to do with the fact that the agent responsible for all the trouble lurks in hot, dark, moist places such as an athlete's changing-room locker. However, the disease affects athletes and nonathletes alike, and plays no favorites. I have seen cases of athlete's foot in infants as young as six months, and in people as old as ninety-five.

A fungus is a very opportunistic agent; a damp towel, a sweaty shoe or sock, or other moist clothing can keep it alive and growing for days, often until it can transfer to a part of the human body. Two of these fungi, *Trichophyton mentagrophytes* and *Trichophyton rubrum,* seek a home in the skin of the foot, and can flourish there because the conditions are perfect for their growth—sweaty, dark, and hot. Once the fungi establish a foothold, they can be tough to dislodge, particularly if the victim delays treatment.

Athlete's foot can attack the healthiest of feet, but only if certain conditions exist. The fungus can hide in a wet piece of clothing or a towel until it comes into contact with a foot that provides a dark, safe haven. For some unknown reason, some people seem to have a built-in immunity to fungal infections, while others need only look at a mildewed towel to wind up with athlete's foot. In health clubs you will see men and women walking around the changing area, the showers, and the pool wearing shower sandals in order to protect their feet from the fungus. Yet they still succumb to the disease. Others walk blithely barefoot through the entire area and never have the slightest hint of a fungal infection. There appears to be a connection between the tendency to contract athlete's foot and fungal nails; these two conditions may constantly reinfect each other.

A few patients have asked me if athlete's foot can spread throughout the body. The family of fungi to which the mentagrophytes belong can make themselves at home anywhere on the body where the proper conditions exist. However, since the leg is neither hot, moist, nor dark compared to the foot or, for example, the groin, it is unlikely that the fungal infection would spread all the way up the leg from a victim's foot. It is possible, however, to contract a *Trichophyton rubrum* infection of hair follicles on the legs.

Most athlete's foot infections occur between the second to the fifth toes. I believe the reason for this involves the so-called soft, or wet, corn that can develop in those areas because of the friction of one toe rubbing against the other. It is not always easy for nonexperts to differentiate between a wet corn and a fungal infection, and in the majority of cases they choose the corn. The unsuspecting sufferer will apply medicated corn pads to the area, but these home remedies contain acids that can burn the skin and destroy its natural defenses against a fungal infection. Not only is the area moist, dark, and hot, but it is now also weakened by the acid, and therefore much more susceptible to a fungal infection. The poor victim may wind up with two problems, if indeed the wet corn did exist.

Although athlete's foot will normally develop first between the toes, it can also initially break out on the sole, particularly on the ball of the foot under the metatarsal heads. Of course, it can also spread rapidly from between the toes to the bottom of the foot, and vice versa.

The infected area itself is well defined by a reddish line around it. Inside the line is whitish, flaking skin where the fungus is growing. It looks like an onion skin peeling, and the discomfort it causes is enough to make you cry. This peeling is nature's way of trying to rid itself of the fungus, but it does not work, because the foreign agent is too tenacious. Anyone who has suffered from athlete's foot can attest to the fact that the condition produces severe itching. Many sufferers complain of a nasty burning sensation as well, particularly when the fungus invades the bottom of the foot. Put all these symptoms together and it becomes much easier to differentiate between a wet corn and athlete's foot.

Slow and Steady Does Not Win the Day

The trick to defeating the athlete's-foot fungus is to catch it early and treat it aggressively. Fortunately, an attack on the fungus does not require expensive medicines and lengthy waits in a doctor's office. Now that you know what causes the problem and how you can identify it, a little common sense and over-the-counter antifungal agents can deal with it before it becomes a major dilemma.

As I have already mentioned, a billion-dollar business has mushroomed out of the need for nonprescription, over-the-counter antifungal medications. Fortunately, most preparations for athlete's foot work quite well when you also eliminate the conditions that the fungi thrive on. The medications come in a variety of sprays, creams, gels, powders, and soaks, and are most effective when applied immediately after the onset of the infection. The area affected by the fungus must also be kept cool, dry, and in the light whenever possible. Those conditions may not always be easy to attain, particularly if you have to be outdoors during the winter months. In warm weather, you ought to be able to stay sockless and barefoot for at least part of the day, although your coworkers at the office may object to your new fashion statement.

Aside from taking all the above steps to defeat the fungus, you should also soak the affected foot in a solution of salt and warm water. The saline solution provides an unappealing atmosphere for the fungus and softens the affected skin, enabling the antifungal preparations applied after the bath to penetrate deeper and act more effectively. The salt and water will also dry the skin somewhat, reducing excess perspiration.

Appropriately enough, the now ubiquitous tea tree oil comes from the folks down under. Australians have apparently used tea tree oil in various forms for years as a remedy for a whole host of skin disorders, including athlete's foot. You may wish to try some, if you can tolerate its somewhat unpleasant odor, although I have no proof of its efficacy in destroying the fungus.

Because the athlete's foot fungus can live for up to fourteen days on the insoles of some shoes, it would be wise, as a preventive measure, to spray all of the shoes you've worn recently with an antifungal preparation, particularly if you have a history of fungal infections.

If you take all the above steps, you have a 75 percent chance of success in treating athlete's foot—if you have not allowed the infection to progress for days. But if the condition has become acute or has been allowed to linger for too long, stronger medications will be required, and they must be dispensed by prescription. A number of these stronger preparations are available in North America, and they are generally quite effective—once again, as long as all the other measures mentioned above are taken.

Partners in Crime

Misery loves company, and the discomfort of athlete's foot can be made worse by simultaneous infection of the area by bacterial agents that love to attack already-weakened sites on the body. Once the fungus has breached the skin, the way is open for all types of alien agents to invade. When a bacterial and a fungal infection flourish in the same place at the same time, it is necessary to use a double-barreled approach to kill them both. Some over-the-counter preparations are both antifungal and antibacterial, and they work quite well. Of course, other steps must also be taken to keep the area dry, cool, and light. If you treat one condition but not the other, a ping-pong situation will develop. First the remaining active infection will pave the way for the return of the other, and then the game will seesaw back and forth until you attack both simultaneously.

Occasionally a third villain enters the fray. When a part of the foot has been attacked by fungi and bacteria over a certain amount of time, the affected area will also become inflamed. If that happens, you must add a third barrel to the shotgun: a topical steroid preparation (a cortisone-type cream) to handle the inflammation. Quite a few drug companies have now combined the three medicines into one topical cream; these are all prescription drugs.

It is important to tackle the inflammation quickly, because the more inflamed the skin, the more hospitable it is to fungal and bacterial infections. Many dermatologists and podiatrists are skeptical about these new three-way creams because steroid creams are contraindicated when a bacterial or fungal infection is present. Medical professionals believe that anti-inflammatory steroid medications actually aid development of a bacterial or fungal infection.

But in severe inflammatory situations the three do work well together, although I prescribe them only when all other treatments have failed.

Return of the Fungi

Most of my patients with athlete's foot naturally want to know if the disease will return once it has been cured. The answer is affirmative. If the same conditions exist that allowed the fungus to attack the foot in the first place, it will strike again, but more often in some people than in others. I mentioned above that some people are more prone to athlete's foot than others. The problem may be one of lifestyle—too much time spent in health-club locker rooms?—but I suspect that it is one of body chemistry. Just as certain people attract mosquitoes and black flies while others do not, many poor souls seem to send out welcome signals to fungi.

If you seem susceptible to fungal infections in general, it would be wise to follow preventive measures. Be careful when you are in public shower and locker-room areas. Take extra care to keep your feet dry and cool, and spray your footwear regularly with antifungal preparations. Try to avoid footwear that has been treated to keep water out, as it also prevents the foot from "breathing," trapping perspiration and creating a warm, moist spot for a fungus to grow. The same applies to wearing anything plastic on the feet, such as sandals or footwear designed to protect against the elements. Plastic footwear has been responsible for increases in fungal infections, particularly in women's feet.

Contact Dermatitis

One of the often baffling mysteries in medicine is what causes contact dermatitis, an inflammation of the skin. The eruption is caused by a foreign agent, but it is neither a fungus nor a bacterium. The foreign agent that causes the condition is a type of chemical or a combination of agents to which you may be allergic. Often the culprit is easy to identify, but at other times it may take days of investigation to pick it out over other suspects. One easy identification would probably be through an article of clothing or footwear made of materials that could produce an inflammation. As an example, many people cannot tolerate black dye next to their skin. Take away the black dye, and the contact dermatitis disappears almost immediately.

But often the problem lies with a chemical, or a combination of chemicals, that may be found in soaps, detergents, perfumes, dyes, glues, or tanning agents that have been used in making a pair of shoes. At other times, a systemic allergic reaction to a drug or a food may make the skin ultrasensitive to things that would not normally irritate it. To compound the puzzle, in clothing, footwear, soaps, lotions, cleaning products, and food there are so many new synthetics and combinations of synthetics on the market today that the search for the allergen becomes like looking for a needle in a haystack. When a medical professional is dealing with contact dermatitis, you can see why he or she often has to play the role of detective.

It can be easier to pinpoint the general cause of contact dermatitis of the foot. If the outbreak occurs specifically when you wear a new pair of shoes or stockings, that item will become the primary suspect. However, it is usually quite difficult to clearly identify what it is in the footwear that is producing the dermatitis. And even when the investigator is lucky enough to identify the chemical involved, how can you, the patient, avoid it in the future when you buy new shoes and stockings? How many shoe or stocking sales personnel know the precise composition of each item they have in their store? Fortunately, many shoe manufacturers have been cooperating with dermatologists and podiatrists, revealing all the materials that have gone into the making of their products. But the list of materials is large, and not all people react adversely to the same chemicals or combinations thereof.

It is easier to identify contact dermatitis on the foot than it is to find the causative agent. It can occur almost anywhere on the foot and is usually a flat rash with red pinpoints. It will erupt fairly quickly after exposure to the irritant or allergen, usually within twenty-four to thirty-six hours, but occasionally sooner if the allergy is a strong one. It is often seen precisely where the strap of a shoe such as a sandal cuts across the bare part of the foot. The area not directly in contact with the shoe will be perfectly normal. The reaction can be compared to the result of a tornado that wreaks havoc over a precisely defined area while leaving adjacent strips of land unscathed.

Once the condition has been diagnosed and the cause discovered, treatment of contact dermatitis is fairly routine. Remove the irritant and try to avoid it in the future. Cortisone-type creams applied to the affected area will help relieve the inflammation. Many of these creams are now widely available over the counter across North America. It also helps to soak the affected foot first in warm, salty water. The soaking opens the pores and allows the cortisone preparation to penetrate deeper under the surface, enhancing its healing capabilities. Moreover, the soaking helps prevent development of a secondary bacterial infection.

Many other types of dermatitis can affect the foot, and while some of them are caused by systemic disorders, others are caused by contact with something to which the person may be allergic. However, contact dermatitis is the most common of the lot, and in this book it would serve no useful purpose to try to list all the others along with their diagnoses, causes, and treatments. My advice to anyone who has a dermatological problem on the foot is to seek the opinion of a specialist, either

a podiatrist or a dermatologist, if the condition does not begin to clear up within a couple of days.

Moles

We turn now to the subject of moles, and straightaway I want to assure you that they are rarely malignant. So you need not cower with fright as you read the following few paragraphs.

A mole is a small, permanent area of pigmentation, or discoloration, on the skin. It is usually brownish in color. Some moles are flat, some are raised; some have hairs growing out of them, others do not. Why they develop in the first place is a moot point; why they change in rare cases from benign to malignant has kept researchers busy for years. However, it has become quite obvious to researchers that overexposure to the harmful rays of the sun is a significant factor in the development of skin cancers in certain groups of people.

We are being told by many medical experts that, unfortunately, the incidence of skin cancers is growing rapidly. Many communities hold on to the mistaken belief that a tanned body is a healthier one. Naturally, the feet are not normally subjected to as much sun exposure as other parts of the human anatomy, so we podiatrists do not see a lot of moles on the foot that can turn into malignant growths.

Moles can appear anywhere on the foot. But when they are on the bottom of the foot or between the toes, they may be more susceptible to irritation. Many experts feel that when a mole is constantly being irritated, it is more likely to present problems than if it sits peacefully unbothered. In any event, only very few moles will ever turn into a *malignant melanoma,* the most lethal form of skin cancer.

When it comes to moles on the feet, I believe that if the possibility of constant irritation exists, they ought to be removed for safety's sake. They can be excised easily in a doctor's office under a local anesthetic, and the site will require only a couple of stitches to close. It is a tiny price to pay for a sound preventive measure.

In general, I believe that all new moles ought to be examined by a doctor. The same applies to any existing mole that suddenly begins growing, changes color, bleeds, or becomes sensitive. It is most important to remember, however, that the odds are strongly in your favor that any mole you have will never cause you any trouble.

Psoriasis

I recall seeing advertisements on television a few years ago for a preparation used to treat psoriasis; it sympathetically referred to the disease as heartbreaking, probably because it can be quite disfiguring to the skin when it is severe. Psoriasis is a skin disease that can apparently be hereditary and results from abnormal overproduction of keratin by the body.

Keratin is a fibrous protein that is essential in the development of healthy skin and nails. Psoriasis can affect either skin or nails, or both at the same time. Although we hear a lot about the disease, psoriasis and psoriatic arthritis affect no more than approximately 2 percent of the North American population. Unfortunately, those few million who do suffer from the disease often have a miserable time, because it is very difficult to treat and it has a nasty habit of recurring.

Psoriasis is characterized by itchy, scaly red patches, and occurs most often on parts of the body where there are bony protuberances, such as the elbow or the knee. As far as the foot is concerned, psoriasis is most likely to be found where a bony area is being constantly irritated. Common sites are pump bumps, bunions, and the soles of the feet.

The disease is not confined to people who are "unwell"; it can strike someone who is otherwise extremely healthy. Stress might be a contributing factor, as might environmental problems, although much research must still be done before the environment can be blamed for either causing or aggravating psoriatic outbreaks. I will, though, ask a patient with psoriasis if he or she has undergone some type of emotional stress during the time in which the condition appeared.

Psoriasis has two interesting features that help in its diagnosis—and diagnosis is not always easy, because the disease can mimic other dermatological disorders, such as dermatitis. One feature is called *Koebner's phenomenon*. If the psoriatic area is traumatized or burned, the lesion will return along with the new growth of skin, which does not happen with most other skin disorders. The second unique aspect of psoriasis is that when the overlying thick, scaly, silvery material is removed from the affected area, there will be pinpoint bleeding underneath it. This is known in the medical world as *Auspitz's sign*.

There is more than one type of psoriasis, unfortunately, and that makes diagnosis of the disease even more complicated. As far as the foot is concerned, one of the most common forms is known as *pustular psoriasis*. It affects the soles of the feet (and the palms of the hands). The affected skin is covered with white, gray, or yellow blisters. The disorder can be confused with various infections, so a culture of the lesions must be taken. If the culture proves to be negative for any type of infection, a diagnosis of pustular psoriasis can be made with a fair degree of accuracy.

A complication of psoriasis is *psoriatic arthritis,* which is definitely a systemic disease rather than a wear-and-tear process. However, only a very small percentage of patients with psoriasis ever contract it. The disease may manifest itself as a mild outbreak on the finger joints, or it can be severe and generalized throughout the body—including the feet—mimicking rheumatoid arthritis. Because of its nature, I believe that cases of psoriatic arthritis ought to be placed in the hands of a rheumatologist for proper evaluation and treatment.

Breaking the Heart of Psoriasis

Psoriasis is not an easy disorder to treat, although researchers have made great strides in the past few years. But until the exact causes of the disease are isolated, we shall have to rely on controlling the symptoms. At present there is no known preventive measure or cure for psoriasis. However, if you search the Internet you will find hundreds of websites devoted to selling you their amazing psoriasis cures.

One of the most effective treatments seems to be to expose the affected area to sunlight. This may be difficult in northern climes in midwinter, but in the warm months of the year, people with psoriasis on their feet ought to get as much sun on the affected area as possible. However, be careful not to wind up with a sunburn. Patients must consult with their dermatologist about the benefits and dangers of unprotected exposure to the sun in the treatment of psoriasis. If sunlight is not readily available, or you prefer not to expose yourself to it, one alternative is ultraviolet-ray therapy. When it comes to controlling psoriasis, ultraviolet light seems to have an effect similar to that of sunlight. But this treatment is not a cure either, and it comes with the same caveat as exposure to sunlight: Too much may contribute to skin cancer.

Some new topical preparations will provide relief, and many more are on the horizon. The cortisone family of skin creams helps, as does the application of coal-tar preparations. Your family physician or dermatologist should be up to date on the latest topical treatment.

If none of the above works, dermatologists can prescribe such alternatives as methotrexate; retinoids; or psoralen drugs plus ultraviolet light (UVA), which is known as PUVA therapy. I tell my patients with stubborn cases of psoriasis to try to keep the disease under control with non-systemic treatments and to be patient. More effective treatments are close at hand.

Sweating It Out

As in the rest of the body, there are sweat glands under the skin of the feet. As well, a normal assortment of bacteria lives on the skin of the feet. When perspiration combines with certain types of bacteria, the result is a bad odor. This odor can be enhanced by environmental conditions such as hot, humid weather and the breathability of shoes and stockings. Some people are not bothered by malodorous feet—their own or those of others. But many are disturbed by their own offensive body odors, and those of people with whom they come in contact. Judging by the number of patients I have who complain about their own foot odor, and if my

patients can be considered a cross section of North American society, the latter are in the majority.

Sweat glands right under the skin secrete the body's nitrogenous wastes. Perspiration is also nature's way of keeping the body's temperature from becoming too high. Thus, when people have a fever, they perspire in an attempt to lower the body temperature to normal. When this heat-reducing perspiration meets up with certain bacteria usually found on the skin, the result can be quite malodorous.

In a sense, then, we are left with a dilemma. How can we allow nature to do what comes naturally, but at the same time prevent unpleasant body odors? I almost always come down on the side of allowing the body to function normally. However, this does not mean that nothing can be done to prevent unappetizing foot odor.

Sweat glands are particularly abundant in the armpits—hence the multibillion-dollar business of underarm antiperspirants and deodorants—and on the soles of the feet. While a variety of products are marketed to control underarm odor, such is not the case for feet. This is why our feet seem to perspire more than most other parts of our body.

There are two primary ways of controlling foot odor. One way is to reduce perspiration by applying an antiperspirant that can be sprayed on, rolled on, or rubbed into the skin. These products, most of which contain aluminum chlorhydrate as their main ingredient, clog the skin pores and prevent sweat from reaching the surface of the skin. Most of them are also perfumed. While reduction of perspiration on the sole of the foot may discourage bacteria from proliferating there, an antiperspirant does not affect bacteria already thriving on the skin surface. Moreover, many people are allergic to the ingredients in the most common antiperspirant products, and may develop nasty rashes where the products have been applied. Most importantly, though, nature is being tampered with. Antiperspirants prevent the natural cooling of the body and natural elimination of waste products. Therefore, if you have a foot-odor problem, I suggest seeking other means of coping.

Another approach is to try to change the type of bacteria that is flourishing on the foot, as some forms of bacteria are far more capable than others of producing unpleasant odors. One method I recommend to my patients is to soak their feet three or four times daily in a saline solution. The solution will destroy certain types of bacteria that cause bad odors. After three or four weeks you may have far fewer odor-producing bacteria on your feet, and the situation may remain that way. An alternative to the saline solution is to apply alcohol, allowing it to dry on the surface of the skin; as it dries, it eliminates odors.

Some people have the misfortune of *hyperhidrosis,* or excessive perspiration on their feet, and this sweat may also be unpleasantly odiferous, a condition known as *bromidrosis.* A combination of the two

conditions is definitely disagreeable, and not that easy to treat clinically. For people suffering from one or both of these conditions, there is a surgical technique known as *sympathectomy.* This procedure involves cutting the part of the nervous system that controls the sweat glands, preventing the glands from reacting to nerve impulses that stimulate perspiration. I am totally opposed to this type of operation, because I strongly believe that nature should not be tampered with in this way.

Along with soaking in a saline solution or applying alcohol, the logical approach to excessively sweaty, odiferous feet is to change shoes and socks as frequently as possible, as much as three or four times a day. This may sound impractical, but until a safe new approach to the problem becomes available, you have little choice, short of what I consider to be uncalled-for surgery. You should wear socks made of natural fibers such as cotton, because they are far more absorbent than synthetic materials. And you should wear shoes that allow the foot to breathe so that moisture has less chance of developing on your feet. Some shoe inserts claim to combat foot odor, and if they help with your particular problem, there is nothing wrong with using them.

Some people have a very different disorder: They do not perspire enough. This condition is known as *anhidrosis,* and it can be either congenital or caused by some other existing disease. A person with anhidrosis will suffer from very dry skin on the bottom of the foot because of lack of necessary moisture. The skin may become so dry as to crack or fissure, particularly in the heel area. If care is not taken to reduce inflammation where the skin has cracked, the fissures may become infected. Nails will also be affected by anhidrosis, and may also begin to crack.

As I have mentioned elsewhere in this book, the best way to treat dry skin on the foot is to apply moisturizing cream twice daily to the affected areas. At night, before going to bed, wrap the affected foot in plastic wrap after the cream has been applied. This will enhance absorption of the cream during the night, because the plastic will seal in whatever perspiration there is on the skin. If there is an infection on the skin or the risk of one, application of an antibiotic cream is recommended along with the moisturizing cream. A pumice stone should be used on the affected areas after bathing or showering to remove dead skin tissue from the foot. This will enhance the growth of new, healthier skin.

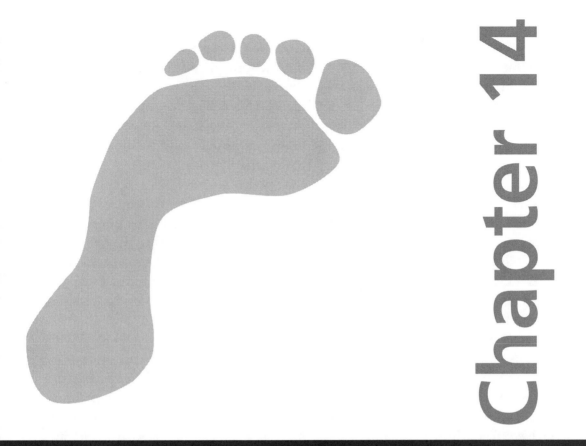

Nail
Problems

Chapter 14: Nail Problems

Nails are horny coverings that protect the tips of the fingers and toes from injury or inflammation. They may also serve as an effective weapon, as anyone who has been scratched by sharp nails can confirm. The forerunners of modern *Homo sapiens* may have used their nails effectively to protect themselves or as a tool to provide food, shelter, and other essentials. This may be why the nail is one of the hardest parts of the human anatomy, and is so durable and potent as a weapon. Although there are differences between fingernails and toenails, they are also quite similar in many respects.

Nails are composed basically of *keratin,* a fibrous protein that grows out of the front part of the top of the toe and slides forward over the nail bed. The root of the nail is also called the *nail matrix,* or *nail growing plate.* The whitish area at the bottom of the nail is the *lunula* (half-moon), and the fold of skin lying directly over the root is the *nail fold.* The layer of skin next to the root is called the *eponychium.* On your fingers you know it as the cuticle.

A healthy nail is clear, with no discoloration anywhere, and a normal nail-growth pattern should follow the contour of the toe. (This is important to remember when cutting your nails.)

Since the nail has no nerve endings, there is no pain directly associated with damage to the nail itself. If the nail is removed, either on purpose or by accident, the discomfort felt comes from the underlying tissue that has been traumatized.

Once that tissue has healed, there will be no discomfort, and the person who lost the nail will be able to function quite normally. This is because the toenail really serves no useful function to modern humans—although many women like to paint them pretty colors as a fashion statement.

One major difference between the toenail and the fingernail is the growth period. Because blood flow to the feet is not as good as to the hands, toenails grow at about one-third the pace of fingernails. It takes about eighteen months for development of a complete toenail.

Numerous things can go wrong with a toenail. Many of these problems produce discomfort and may hinder normal walking. People most commonly affected by nail disorders are those in the over-fifty age group, probably because they are more prone to accidental trauma than most younger adults, and because they have had more years in which to develop and ignore conditions that eventually cause problems.

The most common cause of nail disorders is an insult, accidental or intentional, to a toe: stubbing it, dropping things on it, or having it stepped on by some heavy clod. In most cases it is the big toe that is affected, just because it happens to be a bigger, better target than the others. Some nail disorders are caused by ill-fitting footwear, faulty genetic makeup, or erratic nail-cutting. However, these are all exceptions rather than the norm.

By far the most common of all nail disorders is the ingrown toenail. Let us begin our discussion of what can go wrong with nails by proceeding directly to this painful condition.

Ingrown Toenails

A normal toenail has no "incurvated" sides—that is, sides that grow into the toe itself rather than straight out. An ingrown toenail, on the other hand, breaks the skin of the nail wall and begins to grow into the toe itself. Contrary to popular belief—a belief unfortunately still held by too many medical professionals—ingrown toenails are not normally caused by improper cutting or by wearing shoes that are too tight. Of course, you could definitely make the problem worse by wearing tight shoes or by trying to cut fancy patterns in the toenail. The major cause of ingrown toenails is trauma—somehow injuring the nail. Also, some people have toenails that grow inward instead of straight out for no particular reason. Whatever the cause of the ingrown nail, however, quick attention is necessary to avoid lingering misery and the chance of acute infection.

Ingrown toenails are not only the most common toenail complaint, they also give rise to numerous old wives' tales about how they occur and how they are best treated. We have already examined how they usually develop. But what exactly causes all the concern and discomfort? Well, one of the myths is that the nail itself hurts. But, as I pointed out at the beginning of the chapter, a nail has no nerve endings, so it cannot hurt.

The piece of nail that grows into the side of the nail bed and causes the discomfort is called a *spicule*. Once the spicule punctures and penetrates the skin, the area is open to bacterial growth. This is similar to having any foreign material, such as a sliver of glass or a splinter of wood, penetrate the skin. Once they have found a hospitable home under the surface of the skin, the bacteria have a ready supply of fresh blood, and they can then produce a nasty infection that will have to be treated with antibiotics.

The spicule penetrating the skin is made possible by an incurvated nail that has become curled for one of the reasons mentioned. The incurvation becomes a chronic condition unless the proper treatment is used to permanently end it. Therefore, while it is helpful to treat the ingrown nail and its inherent infection with antibiotics and soaking, to prevent further infection and pain, the root cause of the disorder must be dealt with. I regularly see patients who have been on almost continuous antibiotic therapy for ingrown-toenail infections because they have not had the nail itself properly treated. Considering the potentially harmful effects and costs of frequent antibiotic use, and the decreased effectiveness of such drugs over time, such therapy might be considered to resemble using a bulldozer to kill unwanted pests on your front lawn.

How *Not* to Treat Ingrown Toenails

Many of the myths concerning ingrown toenails revolve around how nails ought to be cut. Many of my patients tell me they have been told that if they cut an ingrown toenail in a V shape in the middle, their problems will be solved. The reasoning behind this idea is that the ingrown nail is too big; hence if a V is cut in the middle, the ends will grow toward the midline of the toe rather than into the sides of the nail wall. This is utter nonsense. You can cut all kinds of artistic patterns into your toenails; if they are incurvated, they will still grow inward.

One elderly female patient told me about her own home remedy for ingrown toenails, a poultice consisting of white bread soaked in milk that has been mixed together with eggs and salt. Apparently the poultice must be applied to the offending toe four times daily if it is to be effective. I do not know how frequently my patient was using it, but when she last came to my office I had to surgically remove her ingrown nail and put her on an antibiotic to clear up the infection. I suggested that in the future she save her poultice for French toast.

The last thing you ought to do is attempt to remove an ingrown nail yourself. I have cautioned you in previous chapters of the dangers of bathroom surgery, and the same warning applies to an ingrown toenail. If you butcher the job—and the odds are excellent that you will—you will still have a spicule stuck under the fold of the skin, and you may develop a very unpleasant infection if one does not already exist.

One old treatment that does have minor merit is to pack the nail groove with cotton. This lifts the nail up somewhat from the nail bed, and it may then grow straight out rather than into the nail wall. However, the chances of success are minimal in the long run, and surgery is by far the treatment of choice.

Surgery for Ingrown Nails

Before I describe the modern surgical techniques for removing an ingrown toenail, I must advise you to avoid an old method that is rather unpleasant. In the old days (and there may be a few doctors around who still use this procedure, hence the warning), the offending part of the nail was excised and the nail-growing plate itself was scraped right down to the toe bone to prevent regrowth of the incurvation. As you can imagine, this is an uncomfortable experience for the patient, who is incapacitated for a week to ten days after the surgery. And, naturally, the risk of postoperative infection is fairly high with such a procedure.

Ingrown nails can be effectively treated with relatively painless "closed" surgery techniques. The primary method is known as *phenol-and-alcohol*—the phenol being an 80 percent carbolic acid solution that is used to kill offending plate-growth cells, and the alcohol a disinfectant to prevent bacterial infection in the area of the surgery.

Despite all the novel treatment techniques that dazzle the medical world, this procedure is still the best treatment method.

The first thing done in the phenol-and-alcohol procedure is to freeze the toe with a local anesthetic. Once the anesthetic has taken hold, the offending part of the ingrown nail is removed with a surgical instrument. Then the nail-growing cells of the incurvated part of the nail are destroyed by applying phenol to the nail bed. The entire procedure takes only a few minutes, and the patient can walk immediately after the operation. Very few patients experience more than a mild throbbing in the area, even after the anesthetic has worn off. In the first few hours after surgery, only about 5 percent of patients from whom I have removed ingrown toenails required a few mild analgesic tablets to relieve minor discomfort; I have never had to prescribe a strong painkiller for any of those patients. I removed an ingrown nail for my coauthor while we were writing this book and, aside from wearing only open-toed sandals for two days, he carried on his normal activities without skipping a beat.

Little postoperative care is required after this minimal incision surgery (MIS) technique, other than soaking the area with warm, salty water three times a day for about a week. For people who may be susceptible to infections, I also prescribe an antibiotic cream to be applied to the site of the surgery. Because no suturing is necessary, there are no stitches to remove, and the procedure is more than 90 percent effective. However, if a spicule does regrow into the side of the nail wall, it will generally happen twelve to eighteen months after the surgery. The new growth can easily be removed using the same phenol-and-alcohol procedure.

One of the major advantages of the phenol-and-alcohol procedure is that the risk of infection is very low. Thus, people with circulatory problems in their lower limbs, such as diabetics, no longer need to fear surgical removal of an ingrown toenail. Moreover, the healing time is much quicker than with old surgical techniques. I have known quite a few people with circulatory problems and ingrown toenails so painful that their lifestyles were adversely affected; in fact, a few had become candidates for amputation of the offending toe. Fortunately, this drastic step is no longer considered, since the risk of infection with MIS is less than 2 percent. The only people who come down with an infection after phenol-and-alcohol surgery are those who refuse to obey the rules of postoperative care. The toe must be soaked at regular intervals *until the area has healed*.

Laser Myths

After an ingrown toenail has been removed, an alternative to application of phenol is the use of a laser to vaporize the nail-growth cells, which prevents regrowth of the incurvation. When this technique was first developed, it was hoped that the laser beam would cause less trauma to the area and even less discomfort to the patient. However, more pain is associated with laser nail surgery, and the recovery period is longer, because the trauma to the area is more severe. Moreover, the laser fails to destroy all the offending nail-growth cells, which means that the ingrown toenail could return to varying degrees. At this time, I do not recommend laser surgery for removal of ingrown toenails.

Rusty Nails

Approximately 75 percent of all the patients over fifty that I see have at least one fungal nail. These *mycotic* nails are really not as bad as they sound, nor are they a result of growing old and "rusty." However, it does seem to be a medical fact that the older you get, the more likely you are to suffer from this disorder, perhaps because a lifetime of neglect of the feet has made you more susceptible. But athletes are also prone to mycotic nails, so if you are over fifty, do not feel that you alone are likely to be plagued by the problem.

Mycotic nails are caused by a tiny microbe—a fungus that requires a dark, moist, fairly hot place in which to flourish. The foot fills the bill perfectly, particularly when you wear shoes for a long time and perspire freely. Of course, another ingredient is required to enable the fungus to settle into a cozy place and grow vigorously until it becomes noticeable. That ingredient is a handy supply of fresh blood under the nail that has been brought to the surface of the

nail bed by some sort of injury to the toe. Given a moist, warm, dark spot and just a tiny supply of fresh blood, the fungus will begin to grow, much as any fungus will grow in a mildew-prone area, such as a damp towel. It will eventually show up on the nail as a yellowish discoloration.

The discoloration of a fungal nail can take up to three or four years to become noticeable. At that time the infected part of the nail will appear to detach itself from the nail bed, but even then it may not cause any significant discomfort.

Treating Fungal Toenails

Of course there have to be a few old wives' tales about treatments for fungal nails. I have heard of people with the disorder who soaked their toes in chlorine detergent, a mixture of vinegar and water, a solution of bleach and laundry detergent, or various similar combinations. None of the above will work a permanent miracle. In fact, probably all the sufferer will wind up with is a clean yellow fungus. You will not have to worry where the yellow went; it will still be there.

If you wish to prevent occurrence of a fungal nail, good hygiene is a must. And if you are unlucky enough to injure a toe, a prophylactic (preventive) application of an antifungal cream or powder is advisable.

Once a fungal nail has been definitely diagnosed, treatment that is relatively simple, painless, and efficient can begin. If the infection is mild, a topical antifungal cream is applied to the affected area two or three times daily for a few months. Fungi usually grow slowly, but they also take a long time to destroy completely, so one must be patient. Fortunately, fungal nails are generally not too uncomfortable, so the wait is not usually that traumatic.

If the fungus has become more obstinate, a stronger cream will work in about 50 percent of cases, though usually only if one nail is involved. These more potent creams are not readily available over the counter, so they will have to be prescribed by a doctor. In the 50 percent of cases where this treatment fails, the foot specialist must proceed to step two.

If topical creams fail to eliminate the fungus, the infected part of the nail may have to be cut out. However, if the nail does not cause the patient any discomfort, I suggest leaving it alone. As with an ingrown nail, excision is done in the doctor's office under a local anesthetic, and it is relatively painless after the operation. Providing that follow-up use of an antifungal cream is continued until the area is completely healed and free of any signs of fungal infection, the success rate for this operation is about 80 percent. About 20 percent of the difficult cases defy both topical cream treatment and excision of the offending nail. In such cases I completely remove the offending nail-growing cells, using the same technique as for an ingrown nail.

There is also another treatment, which is systemic rather than topical. This is the antifungal pill, which was developed during the past ten years to combat toenail fungi. As with most medications taken internally, the pills have side effects, some of which make practitioners very careful when prescribing them. Prescribing medication is always a risk-versus-reward scenario, and the doctor has to worry whether the complications of the drug are outweighed by the benefit of getting rid of the nail fungus. If it is suggested that you might need to take these pills, make sure that your doctor explains to you their adverse effects. And be wary of media advertisements for such pills. These drugs can seriously affect your health!

These medications kill the fungus at the nail-growing cells, so it can take from twelve to eighteen months for patients to see the results, even though they take the drug for only three months. A year to a year-and-a-half is the normal length of time required for new nail growth to completely replace the fungal nail. These drugs are about 80 percent effective, so a cure is not guaranteed. They do have fewer side effects than earlier antifungal drugs, but caution must be used, since even those side effects can be dangerous.

Crazy Nails

I am not referring here to weird and wonderful fingernail coverings, but to certain toenail problems that come under the general heading of *onychogryphosis*. This medical term is used to describe a thick, distorted nail that has become abnormal for a variety of reasons, most often traumatic injury. A less common cause is years of constantly wearing shoes that do not fit properly. The problem is one of damage to the nail bed and the nail-growing cells. My theory is that if a normal nail has been injured, the nail plate becomes damaged, and the cells respond by growing a thicker nail to protect the nail-growing area and the nail bed. This is not an accepted medical fact, but it seems logical to me.

One of the most common of distorted, or gryphotic, nail problems is the ram's horn. In this case, the nail spirals toward one side of the toe, taking on the appearance of a sheep's curly horn. A toenail can also take on other crazy shapes if the toe has been traumatized. In all cases the treatment is roughly the same.

Treating the Crazy Nail

Once the damage has been done, the only treatment that appears to work with any degree of success is excision of the entire offending nail using the phenol-and-alcohol technique. However, other, more conservative steps can be tried first. The reason that people seek relief from gryphotic nails is the same as for fungal nails: They can become painful at times, and they are unpleasant to look at. Yet some people are so embarrassed by the appearance of their distorted toenails that they avoid treatment altogether, even when they are in pain.

The first conservative step I take with patients who do seek a remedy is to grind, smooth, and trim the gryphotic nail, and then have the patient apply moisturizing creams nightly to the affected area. The creams will keep the nail soft, and therefore easier to trim. A concurrent step is to persuade the patient to wear shoes that fit properly. Wearing proper footwear will relieve pressure on the offending toe and prevent the situation from worsening.

If the deformed nail causes pain or is too unsightly for the patient to tolerate, and if conservative treatments do not work, the problem will most likely have to be treated surgically, using the phenol-and-alcohol method. As I mentioned above, this is the only treatment that seems to be reasonably successful.

The Psoriatic Nail

The psoriatic nail is caused by psoriasis in the skin around the nail, and involves the nail bed where the nail-growing cells are located. Psoriatic nails generally become thick and yellow, and whitish longitudinal lines often run down the nail. The top layer of a psoriatic toenail will be very brittle. However, if you were to remove that top layer you would find that the underlying portion of the nail is soft and very flaky.

Psoriasis of the nail is most difficult to treat. Some cortisone creams will help a little, but they do not offer a permanent cure. I hesitate to go into great detail about treatments, because I believe that anyone with a psoriatic condition, even a psoriatic nail, should be under a doctor's care rather than relying on home remedies.

I do not recommend surgical removal of a psoriatic nail. This is because the skin around and under the nail tends to become more prone to psoriasis after nail-removal surgery, and therefore will probably be more uncomfortable than the original affected nail.

Good Nail Hygiene

Now that we have discussed the major nail problems, let us end this chapter by summarizing what you can do to keep your nails from causing you trouble.

First, cut your toenails to align with the contour of your toes. If you cut your nails straight across, the jagged corners can catch on socks or pantyhose and can even irritate adjacent toes. If your toenails have rough edges, use a nail file to smooth them. Do not dig out the corners of your nails. You may make them bleed, and that could result in fungal and/or bacterial infection.

To prevent an ingrown nail from pushing deep into the skin, try using a mild commercial acid-based preparation that acts to soften the skin (not the nail) and/or a softening cream or moisturizer. A pharmacist can assist you with the purchase. However, be careful if the nail is incur-

vated; the acid will not help much, and using too much of the solution could cause burns and/or infections, just like indiscriminate use of a corn pad or callus pad.

If you have been told to soak your toes for a nail problem, I recommend using a saline solution—for example, one teaspoon of Epsom salts to one quart of warm water.

If you have a suspected infection in a nail area that over-the-counter antibacterial or antifungal creams or powders do not help, get medical attention quickly to prevent further infection, particularly if the offending area is red, swollen, or discharging. Bathroom surgery for any condition is, of course, a definite no-no. This applies particularly to anyone with a circulatory problem or diabetes.

If you injure a toe slightly and notice some bleeding under the nail, immediate application of an antifungal agent is advisable to prevent a fungal infection. If the nail itself is badly damaged by an accident, I recommend immediate medical attention to prevent complications such as those we have discussed in this chapter.

If you have trouble cutting your toenails properly, I strongly urge you to have a podiatrist or chiropodist take care of them for you, or teach you how to care for them properly yourself. Finally, if you have a circulatory problem and develop an abnormal toenail condition, do not play around with it yourself—and do not ignore it!

Chapter 15

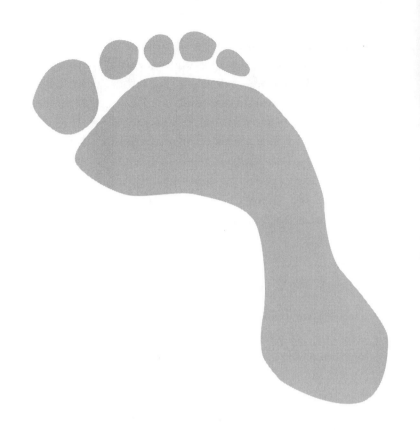

In Search of a Shoe That Fits

According to Roman historians, Julius Caesar was determined to make his foot soldiers travel farther and faster, and he reckoned that a change in footwear might improve the speed and agility of his fighting men. He decided to experiment with the heel height of their boots. Caesar's best scientific minds eventually concluded that the soldiers marched faster and lasted longer on their feet without tiring when their heels were about one inch high. Caesar's experiments may have been the first scientific studies to determine the most comfortable shoe to wear, but they were certainly not the last.

Analysis of the average person's gait has convinced running-shoe manufacturers that the Roman scientists were basically correct—one inch is the optimum heel height for shoes for the average person. Today, unfortunately, platform shoes are again fashionable. *Et tu,* platform! This ridiculous footwear can cause severe ankle and leg fractures when the unwitting wearer falls off them. If only shoe manufacturers would pay attention to that fact—or perhaps personal injury lawyers ought to take note. Although wearing improper shoes may not be the primary cause of foot miseries in modern society, it can certainly aggravate existing conditions, as well as cause quite a few on its own.

I have divided this chapter into two parts: The first section deals with shoes in general, particularly women's shoes; the second with athletic footwear specifically. As you will learn, if I ruled the world, I would insist on the wearing of running shoes most of the time—except when the wearer is engaged in some physical activity that requires other athletic footwear or specialty items such as skates or ski boots.

One of the problems with footwear selection in general is that some of the people selling shoes for men, women, and children know absolutely nothing about feet or biomechanics. They know only about sales commissions and/or styles. Would you have a suit or dress fitted by someone who knew nothing about tailoring? If not, then why would you allow a person who knows nothing about feet to fit you with a pair of shoes? I always tell my patients who wear ill-fitting shoes to make sure that the salesperson fitting them knows something about feet and the footwear the store sells. If that salesperson cannot satisfactorily answer questions about the size and shape of shoes appropriate for them or about inherent biomechanical problems in certain styles, they are advised to seek another salesperson—or another store.

The Shoemakers

Up until the Industrial Revolution, shoes were made by a local shoemaker who tailored his footwear to fit his customers. All shoemakers had their own designs and types of footwear—boot, shoes, etc.—that were their trademarks, but what most of them had in common was their ability to provide comfort for their customers. But now footwear is mass-produced to fit the average foot, not the individual foot. Moreover, the shoe manufacturers' major concern is, logically enough, turning a profit.

Today shoes are sold on the basis of fashion design; it seems that modern men and women are willing to sacrifice comfort when it comes to shoe selection. This sad fact may be good for my business, but I also find it frustrating because, although I can make my patients' feet feel better, I can't keep them that way if they refuse to wear proper shoes. Actually, I am being a bit unfair; many people would wear shoes that fit them properly if only they could find them.

The typical manufacturer of shoes makes sizes that could properly fit 75 percent of the population. This means that about 25 percent of the people who wear fashionable shoes are wearing ill-fitting footwear. Many manufacturers also leave out the half-sizes to cut their costs. So, if your foot is not of average size, you may have great difficulty finding the proper shoe for your foot in the size you need and at a price you can afford. As a result, you may settle for a shoe that does not quite fit properly.

Some shoe manufacturers do make all sizes and widths, but they generally offer fewer and less stylish models because they are usually small enterprises, without a large design component. Moreover, even when their shoes might be considered fashionable, their output is so small relative to the demand that very few shoppers can find them.

Men are slightly better off than women, perhaps because the style of men's shoes does not vary much from year to year. That may be because heel height is not a major factor in the design of most men's shoes, so less can be done to change the style. Older men seem to prefer the brogue or wingtip style of shoe, possibly because—as one of my first male patients told me years ago—brogues most resemble the footwear they had to wear in the armed forces, and they like them because they provide the best support. Whatever the reason for the popularity of certain men's shoe styles, manufacturers can produce more shoes in odd sizes, knowing that they will eventually be sold—if not this month or this year, then next month or next year. Similarly, shoe retailers will not panic when men's shoes do not sell immediately, because they know the merchandise will eventually be purchased.

Victims of Fashion

Women with uncommon shoe sizes are not as lucky as men, because fashion plays a much greater role in the manufacture of women's footwear. This year's style may not reappear for years, so why should the manufacturer produce extra quantities in odd sizes, and why should shoe retailers stock them when they might be stuck forever with unwanted inventory?

An overwhelming majority of the 25 percent of women who have uncommonly sized feet have the same problem: a narrow heel and a broad forefoot. To produce a shoe to fit this kind of foot, the manufacturer must make a *combination-last* shoe. The last refers to the form on which the shoe is shaped, and the result can be compared to the frame of an automobile. There are two basic types of lasts, straight and curved, which is important, particularly if you have a foot problem. The two things to remember are that the last should conform to the basic shape of your foot, and that most shoes are single-lasted. A combination-last shoe requires greater production time and costs, and it is not as easy to make this type of shoe appear as stylish as a single-lasted shoe.

A woman with a narrow heel and a broad forefoot may have, for example, a heel width of AA and a forefoot width of B. Shoes with an AA heel and a B forefoot are not easy to find, and when they do reach the stores, as I have mentioned, they are gobbled up quickly by the smart early-bird shoppers. Until shoe manufacturers begin mass-producing stylish products with combination lasts, women who want fashionable shoes that fit them comfortably will have to either shop with an eagle eye or settle for a poorer fit. Unfortunately, too many women in this position opt for style over comfort, and eventually they pay the price in foot problems. Today, two or three manufacturers produce semi-custom-designed women's fashion shoes that are sold in a retail setting; time will tell whether this will solve the majority of the problems.

Unbelievably, the newest rage in the fashion hotspots is "plastic surgery" on feet to give the owners the exact feet they always wanted! Let's not concern ourselves with the shoe fitting the foot; let's cut the foot to fit the shoe! I discuss the negative aspects of this surgery in Chapter 16.

The Right Fit

Another factor to consider when purchasing a new pair of shoes is the sizing used by particular manufacturers. Every shoe manufacturer uses a different last, just as every carmaker has a different standard body frame. And, like automobile manufacturers, shoe producers also make many different models. So, for example, the same shoe producer can make a variety of size 9 shoes from totally different lasts. The result is a totally different fit for each model.

If a person tells me that he or she is a perfect size 8½, I say, "Nonsense," because there are no perfectly consistent size 8½ shoes. One manufacturer's size 8½ is another's size 8 or 9. Keep this in mind when you are shopping for new footwear, and do not hesitate to go up or down a half-size if your normal fit suddenly seems abnormal. In all probability your foot has not changed dimensions; you are most likely trying on a different model of shoe, possibly from a company whose products you have never tried before.

Shoe manufacturers and consumers seem to have forgotten—or choose to ignore—the fact that the primary functions of a shoe are to cover and to protect the foot. (The makers of athletic shoes tend to be exceptions. I will discuss such footwear in detail later in this chapter.) If we lived in warm climates and spent all our waking hours strolling along the beach or walking on soft grass, we would not even require footwear. We tend to forget that our ancestors in warmer climes never covered their feet, and neither do certain cultures even today.

What Shoes to Buy

When you shop for a new pair of shoes, remember that price has no relationship to comfort, unless you are seeking modern running shoes or very soft leather shoes that allow your foot added flexibility. There are also three things that you must take into consideration besides size. The first is flexibility: Does the shoe allow your foot to bend where it is supposed to bend? The second is stability: Does the shoe keep the foot positioned properly during the gait cycle to lessen the possibility of a biomechanical fault? The third is shock absorption: Does the shoe provide sufficient cushioning to take undue stress off the foot during the stance phase of the gait cycle?

Today, many shoe manufacturers are producing "comfort shoes" that attempt, with fair success, to combine a modicum of style with the attributes of athletic shoes. Shoes from these manufacturers—for example, Rockport, Mephisto, Easy

Spirit, and Ecco—are available in many retail footwear and athletic goods stores. I have even seen a commercial that shows members of a women's basketball team playing in this type of "dress" shoe. Athletic footwear companies—for example, Nike, Reebok, and Adidas—are also marketing their versions of the comfort shoe.

The one type of shoe that comes closest to meeting all three criteria noted above is the modern running shoe, which has been able to combine flexibility, stability, and shock absorption without sacrificing too much of any quality. This is one type of shoe that tends to improve as the price increases, although running shoes are not nearly as expensive as high-fashion shoes. Comfort shoes are decent walking shoes that sacrifice a little of the above-noted criteria but still offer excellent quality and, for many, preferable styles. But they cannot provide the same amount of flexibility, stability, and cushioning as a running shoe.

I understand why most people are unable to wear running shoes all the time, although businesspeople and fashion models often wear them to work and then switch into fashionable footwear at the office. However, if you have a lower-back, hip, or knee problem, you ought to consider wearing running or walking (comfort) shoes whenever you can. They help compensate for biomechanical faults and provide much better cushioning than most other shoes. If you cannot wear such footwear most of the time, keep in mind that rubber or crepe soles provide better shock absorption than other types of soles.

Children's Shoes

Bad footwear habits begin in childhood, often as a result of parental misguidance. Two problems come to the fore in contributing to children wearing the wrong shoes at the wrong time in their development. The first is that old ideas die hard, and children are often forced into the type of shoes that their parents had to wear when they were the same age. I am speaking of those inflexible oxfords that parents used to think were essential for arch support. The second problem is that children often become fashion-conscious at too early an age, and they want uncomfortable shoes that look pretty or are the "in" footwear. That may be acceptable if they want a good pair of athletic shoes that a sports hero is wearing, but not if the latest fad is a spike heel worn by some female celebrity.

There is no proof that any shoe except a well-constructed running shoe is good for a child with normal feet. And most children with foot abnormalities are better off with running shoes and orthotics than heavy, unyielding oxfords. If corrective shoes are required, they must be prescribed by a specialist. Do not allow a shoe salesperson to talk you into any type of shoe inserts for your child. As I mentioned previously, a child's foot may be harmed by correcting a fault that does not require immediate attention. If you are at all concerned about your child's feet and footwear, have that child examined by a specialist, not by a shoe salesperson who may recommend an unnecessary, and potentially harmful, shoe insert.

As far as adolescents are concerned, they often wear running shoes while at school or play because they are the most comfortable. However, young girls can develop the bad habit of wearing shoes with three-inch and higher heels before they have finished growing, and that can cause problems, particularly with their knees (see Chapter 8). Although I am against high-heeled shoes in general, I believe they are particularly harmful to young girls.

Adult Shoes

My comments on the evils of high-heeled shoes apply equally to adults. The human body was not designed to walk on three-inch or four-inch heels, which produce severe anatomical distortions and can result in orthopedic problems from the lower back down to the feet. Back specialists agree that high-heeled shoes are one major cause of backaches in women. High-heeled shoes put abnormal stress on the back of the leg, the knees, and the lower back, and, if worn regularly, result in shortened Achilles tendons. They also put tremendous stress on the forefoot, which is probably being squeezed by a tight toe-box as well. There is little I can add to what I have already said about the perils of high heels, except to appeal again to women to avoid them if possible.

Chapter 15: In Search of a Shoe That Fits

Some heels are even higher than just high. I am referring to spike-heeled shoes that are at least four inches high and have sharply pointed toe-boxes. The only nice thing I can say about these shoes is that they are good for the podiatric business. They do everything bad for the foot that three-inch, high-heeled shoes with pointed toe-boxes do, only much worse.

Slingback shoes have a strap in the rear to hold the foot in place, and are generally no more than two inches in heel height. Although they provide good breathability for the foot in warm weather, they offer no stability in the heel and provide little shock absorption for the foot. However, they are reasonably flexible and comfortable, and much less damaging for the average foot than higher-heeled shoes. An advantage of many slingback shoes is that the heel width can be adjusted by the strap.

The negative-heel shoe ("Earth" shoes) became popular during the hippie era and was advertised as being "natural." But there was nothing natural about the lower back and leg pains that they caused. Negative-heel shoes force the Achilles tendon to over-stretch, which in turn causes muscles and tendons all the way up into the lower back to overextend. They also produce an abnormal stance phase in the gait cycle because they force the heel to remain on the ground for too long. This leads to all sorts of bio-mechanical foot faults. Fortunately, in spite of attempts to revive it, the negative-heel shoe is basically history; let's hope it stays that way.

Wooden shoes, or clogs, are very popular in certain societies because they provide decent metatarsal and longitudinal arch support, although they are inflexible and do not offer much shock absorption. The shoe itself mimics an arch support, and if you overpronate it will provide some stability.

Sandals are popular in warm climates because they allow the feet to breathe comfortably and therefore remain reasonably dry and cool. But very few sandals provide adequate stability or shock absorption, so they are not recommended for people with lower limb problems. However, I am now able to offer my patients sandals with prescription orthotics built right into the shoe, although they are expensive.

High boots are quite fashionable in the winter. It is difficult to rate them as a group, because heel heights vary considerably. The rule of thumb is that they should be treated as high-heeled shoes if the heels are above two inches. The only other thing to mention about such boots is their lack of breathability. Unless they are lined, they are not going to keep your feet that warm, but they will reduce circulation of air around the lower extremities, and your feet and lower legs may actually feel a bit clammy.

As I mentioned earlier, men's footwear is not normally as hard on the feet as are women's shoes. The main concerns in men's shoes are proper fit, adequate room in the toe-box, decent shock absorption, stability, flexibility, and lacing that does not pinch the nerves on top of the front part of the foot. Men who are not vain rarely wear shoes with heels that are higher than one inch. If they do, they will have problems similar to those of women who wear them regularly.

The Geriatric Shoe

Older people often have more trouble with their feet than their juniors. Therefore, it is important for them to wear the proper footwear. And because they often have circulatory problems in their lower limbs, they have to keep their feet warm in cold weather to prevent frostbite or immersion foot (chilblain).

It is imperative for seniors to find shoe salespeople who know how to fit shoes and can offer advice on what stockings to wear in different weather. My advice to them is to wear good running shoes as often as possible, because they provide the best overall protection and comfort, particularly when used for walking and exercising. There is no reason why a healthy older person should not be able to enjoy a daily constitutional in comfort, without any footwear concerns.

Seniors can now find in specialty stores shoes that are designed specifically for geriatric problems such as swelling and nonoperable disorders (because of systemic diseases such as diabetes and poor cardiovascular function) like hammer toes, bunions, and plantar-flexed metatarsal heads. These shoes are made of softer materials, have much deeper toe-boxes, and

provide better support. They may also have extra cushioning in the forefoot to make up for loss of the fat pad under the sole. Seniors with this painful problem should try to find these special shoes, or at least buy shock-absorbing inserts to fit into their regular shoes.

Finally, I'd like to take to task a new industry that has developed by selling the idea to older people that, for those who walk for exercise, the walking shoe is the ultimate footwear. Nonsense! A good running shoe is *much* better for walking than a so-called walking shoe. Running shoes provide superior shock absorption, greater flexibility and motion control, and better breathability, and are usually made of better materials. Although walking shoes are a big improvement over other types of footwear, they cannot hold a candle to the excellent running shoes being manufactured today.

If the Shoe Fits . . .

A final piece of advice I want to give is about trying on shoes, no matter what their style. I have often heard patients say that they have to break in their shoes, that their shoes are never comfortable when they buy them, but gradually give until they fit the feet. The problem with this theory is, if they do not fit at first, what damage are they doing to your feet during the breaking-in period? And why do so many people who argue that their shoes have to be broken in have foot problems?

If a shoe does not feel good when you first try it on, don't buy it! That shoe is obviously not right for your foot—and it most likely never will be. Conversely, if a pair of shoes feels fine at first but then becomes uncomfortable, don't continue to wear them. You may not feel that you got your money's worth, but you have to accept the fact that the shoes are not right for your feet, and chalk up the disappointment to experience.

Athletic Footwear

Athletic-footwear companies are playing a major role in lower-limb injury prevention, not necessarily for altruistic reasons, but because the market is so competitive these days that they have to stay a step ahead of the field. The industry is spending millions of dollars each year to produce the perfect shoes to give different athletes ultimate performance. Just as automobile racers rely on certain tires for a competitive edge, so athletes rely on footwear to give them an advantage over the competition. Certain athletic activities require different types of shoes because stresses and ground surfaces may differ. And, since every athlete has a different foot, a single shoe last may suit one but not another. The end result is that, except for children who are not playing a specific sport, there is no longer any such thing as the all-purpose sneaker or running shoe.

All this competitiveness and research has led to a much better product for the athlete, but usually at a higher price per pair of shoes. However, let me assure you that when it comes to athletic shoes, you do get what you pay for, almost all the time. The major problem for the athletic consumer today is how to choose the proper pair of shoes from among the proliferation of models and manufacturers.

Because athletic shoes today are sport-specific, you would be well advised to find a store that carries a wide variety of shoes for all sorts of activities and that employs sales personnel who are familiar with the merchandise and the needs of specific athletes. If you have a definite biomechanical problem in your lower limbs, you would be wise to consult first with a podiatrist who is an expert in sports medicine. Then you will know better exactly what type of shoe to look for. You must also take into consideration the type of surface on which you will be exercising. Different terrains, court surfaces, or playing fields will call for different types of shoes. Avoid buying the best-looking or highest-priced athletic shoe without taking the above into consideration. If you have any doubts at all, keep shopping until you find a knowledgeable salesperson. Remember, although a certain shoe may feel okay when you try it on in the store, it may be totally inadequate for your needs when you are exercising.

The three major factors to consider when purchasing athletic shoes are, as for nonathletic shoes, cushioning (shock absorption), stability, and flexibility. Recent developments in designing and manufacturing these shoes have resulted in footwear that is far superior to that of twenty years ago, and their increased stability, flexibility, and shock absorption provide more comfort than any other type of shoe made today. That is why it is not unusual to see business executives, both male and female, wearing running shoes to work, switching to regular shoes only when they reach their offices. Let's take a closer look at a typical modern running shoe to find out exactly why it helps protect the feet and legs from injury.

Cushioning (Shock Absorption)

Most of the shock on a foot is absorbed through the midsole that spans the length of the shoe (see Figure 15.1). The thickness of the highly resilient material used for cushioning is generally approximately one inch at the heel and a third to half an inch at the forefoot. The additional thickness at the heel allows for the extra stress created during the heel-strike phase of the gait cycle. It reduces the risk of trauma to the

Figure 15.1. Anatomy of a running shoe

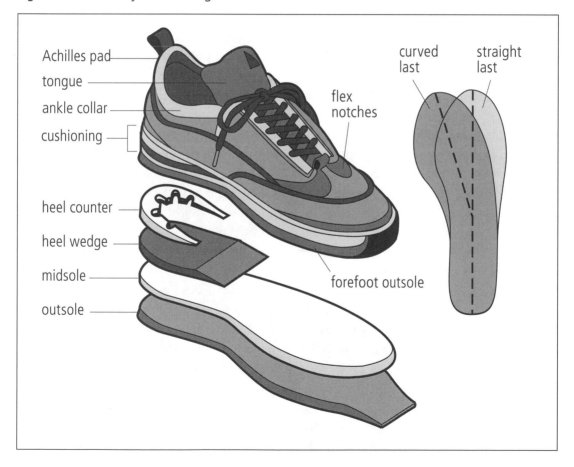

heel and to the Achilles tendon. Some shoes also have a built-in cushioning system on the outer sole, where contact is made with the ground during the running stride. This space-age cushioning has certainly cut down the number of traumatic overuse injuries to runners' feet, particularly in the heel area. Depending on the make and style of the shoe, the cushioning in today's athletic footwear can range from air to water to gel.

Stability

The modern running shoe also features high-tech extra stability devices to improve foot control. The more foot control the shoe offers, the less chance there is of wear-and-tear disorders caused by stressful, repetitive motions. Because of great improvements in the materials used, running shoes can now provide better stability with more motion control. Many insoles have a material on the outside that is harder than in the middle, to help prevent rolling of the foot when it strikes the ground. Much better control of torsion (twisting from the front of the shoe to the back) helps prevent biomechanical abnormalities.

Although running shoes are constantly improving, manufacturers are still having trouble providing maximum stability without sacrificing cushioning properties, and vice versa. Also, stability is often traded off for a lighter-weight shoe, as many runners would rather have the comfort of a lighter shoe than the added stabil-

ity. If they do not have any foot problems, they can easily get away with this trade-off.

A lot of shoe manufacturers have combined different densities of foam in the midsole to provide greater rigidity in various areas. Firm internal and external heel counters have also been added in some shoes for more rearfoot control. The plethora of new designs is seemingly endless, as manufacturers vie for a healthy share of the athletic-footwear market. In the long run, the winner will be the athlete, as the competition among manufacturers will ensure continuous improvements in these shoes.

One of the most important factors determining stability in a shoe is the last. As I mentioned earlier, the last refers to the shape of the sole, and can be compared to the frame of an automobile before the chassis is mounted on it. The two most common types of lasts are straight and curved, and a few rules govern the choice of type. First, if the shape of your foot is basically straight and if you have a low arch, the straight-lasted shoe is best for you, because it offers more support on the inside of the foot and will help prevent you from overpronating, enabling you to minimize overpronation injuries.

If your foot is slightly curved, if you have a higher than normal arch when standing, or if you have been diagnosed as having a rigid foot, you will probably feel more comfortable in curve-lasted shoes. These shoes offer more cushioning but still retain rearfoot stability. People who oversupinate often find that curve-lasted shoes are much better for them, because the shape of their feet and that of the shoe are compatible.

If you are uncertain as to which type of last to get, you might want to seek expert advice before buying your next pair of athletic shoes. Many runners, though, can tell whether they require a straight or a curved last just by walking in the shoes for a few minutes.

Flexibility

Flexibility in a running shoe is necessary to take excessive strain off the muscles in the lower leg while you are running. Most flexible shoes today provide better shock absorption than inflexible ones, with little loss in stability. When shopping for a pair of running shoes, you should try bending the shoe in half at the midfoot area. If this cannot be done easily, try another pair. You can also determine flexibility by examining the *forefoot outsole patterns* on the bottom of the shoe and looking for *flex notches* on the sides. These patterns and notches are not there for aesthetic purposes; they are designed to provide the required flexibility—most importantly, in the area of the metatarsal heads and toes.

Other Footwear Factors

There are a few other factors to consider when purchasing a running shoe, particularly the breathability of the shoe, and especially in the upper, forefoot part. You do not want too much moisture to be trapped inside your shoe, as fungi and blisters thrive in hot, moist areas. You will also want to know what sort of traction the outer sole provides. You do not want to be slipping and sliding when you are running.

Is the shoe you are choosing light in weight, but still able to provide the stability you need? Generally speaking, the lighter the shoe, the less stability it has to offer. Is there cushioning around the ankle that includes an Achilles pad (see Figure 15.1), to prevent irritation to this area and consequent skin eruption? Is the tongue of the shoe padded to prevent the laces from pressing on the top of the foot? Finally, is there a removable inner sole in case you must add prescribed orthotics?

Racket Sports and Aerobics Shoes

Many of the remarks I have made above refer specifically to running shoes, which are designed to support a foot that is constantly moving forward. These types of shoes are not designed for repeated bouncing up and down on one's toes or for quick lateral movements. Sports activities that require a lot of lateral movements necessitate a shoe that provides more lateral support for the foot. And many activities, such as aerobics, place stresses on the forefoot, so they require shoes with additional shock-absorptive qualities in the front.

Racket sports involve repeated, quick, stop-and-go movements in all directions. Running shoes do not provide for such movements, particularly because of the added cushioning in their heels and a lack of lateral stability in the forefoot. Raised heels make the back part of the foot less stable, and quick lateral movements can result in sprained ankles. So if you wish to minimize the risk of a lower-limb injury while playing racket sports, buy shoes specifically designed for such activities. The court is no place for a running shoe. And shoes for racket sports are now becoming surface-specific, with tennis shoes for clay surfaces as well as for Tartan (synthetic polyurethane) or asphalt courts.

Many problems make foot and leg injuries the constant companions of aerobics exercisers. The exercises are usually done on a fairly hard surface. Exercisers may spend a lot of time on their toes and, depending on the instructor's routines, moving laterally. Lateral movement is particularly accentuated when aerobics are combined with dancing, as in dancercise. So an aerobics exerciser must have a shoe that combines added forefoot cushioning with flexibility and stability.

Manufacturers of aerobics shoes are continuing their research to develop the perfect product, and for people who are not prone to leg and foot problems and who exercise on surfaces that have some resilience, the modern aerobics shoe is fine. But if you are constantly plagued by problems such as shin splints or are forced to exercise on hard, unyielding surfaces, I recommend that you stick to good running shoes, because you require cushioning that even the best aerobics shoe cannot yet offer. Definitely avoid wearing a racket-sports shoe for aerobics, because this type of shoe is made for lateral mobility and fails to provide adequate flexibility and the shock absorption required for aerobic exercising.

If you do a lot of step aerobics, you require shoes that grip better and have more flexibility in the front part of the foot. Because of the pull on the Achilles tendon, stair-climbers need exercise shoes that have higher heels, particularly if they have a history of Achilles problems due to a shortened tendon.

Hiking is also a popular aerobic pastime these days. Stability is very important for hikers because they are constantly walking or climbing on uneven surfaces. High-top hiking shoes provide much of the additional stability they require.

Other Sports Footwear

A few years ago the major manufacturers of athletic shoes began branching out. High-top basketball-type shoes became popular, particularly when they were advertised by hoop superstars. Now, not only do the manufacturers make running, aerobics, and racket-sports shoes, they also produce footwear for every imaginable athletic activity and for all types of surfaces. Baseball players, for example, now have shoes designed specifically for use on artificial turf to protect them from injuries such as turf toe. It is not feasible for this book to discuss in detail every type of sports shoe on the market today. I can only advise athletes to consult with their trainer, coach, or a knowledgeable sports-shoe salesperson, and to try on the models available for their specific sport to determine the best possible shoe to buy. The rule should be that if shoes do not feel comfortable during the physical activity, do not wear them at all. The lower limbs could be injured and overall performance will suffer if the shoes do not fit comfortably. Many of the major athletic-footwear stores now provide various surfaces on the premises to allow customers to try out the shoes under typical conditions for their type of activity.

Some athletes worry about whether they should buy all-leather shoes or shoes that are half leather and half nylon mesh. All-leather shoes are more durable, obviously, but they are also heavier. The half-and-half shoes are lighter and provide greater breathability for the foot. You must weigh the trade-offs for yourself and buy the shoes in which you feel the most comfortable. There is no noticeable difference in performance between the two types.

The Asphalt Jungle

Humans may be the only animals that do most of their running and walking on hard, man-made surfaces like concrete and asphalt. Of course, I am referring to modern man, particularly people who live and work in urban areas and rely on roads and sidewalks for level surfaces on which to exercise or get back and forth. This is a shame, because grass or a level dirt path would provide far more shock absorption than pavement. In most urban areas, a nice level path of grass or dirt to run on is difficult or impossible to find, so runners train on sidewalks or roadways.

It is imperative that the surface on which you run at least be free of potholes and sudden, sharp dips, and not be overly canted (sloped). One bad step on an uneven surface could result in a severe ankle or knee-joint injury. As well, runners often neglect to take into serious consideration the pounding to which their bodies are being subjected as they run on hard surfaces. The added shock of a hard landing on the foot accentuates biomechanical foot faults, and can lead to injuries such as stress fractures. The most important thing runners can do is wear running shoes that provide the best shock absorption. Extra shock-absorbing material in running shoes will considerably reduce the jarring forces to which the body is subjected with each stride.

The floors on which aerobic exercises are often done have also been blamed by sports-medicine specialists for development of problems caused by excessive shock to the foot and leg. One common injury is shin splints. Fortunately, good fitness clubs have recognized the problem and have sought more resilient surfaces to install in their exercise areas. They have found that not only do their members remain more injury-free, but their instructors miss fewer classes because of shin splints and other overuse problems. As I mentioned above, if you do aerobic exercises on a very hard floor, you should wear running shoes, because they provide the best shock absorption for your feet. And, as I noted in Chapter 12, switching to low-impact and step aerobics will dramatically reduce the number of stress fractures, shin splints, and knee and iliotibial band injuries.

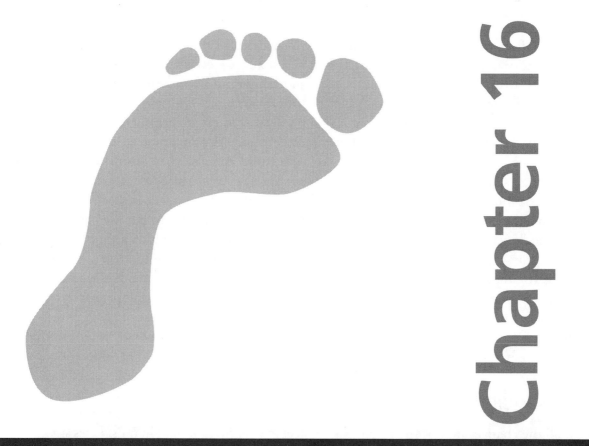

Chapter 16

The Latest in Noninvasive Care and Foot Surgery

Chapter 15: The Latest in Noninvasive Care and Foot Surgery

As I mentioned in the Introduction, dramatic improvements in foot care have been made over the past decade. Advancements in diagnostic techniques have been a major achievement: Computer technology has been updated to analyze the biomechanics of a person's gait, and scans are increasingly available to unearth foot disorders that might otherwise go unnoticed or be misdiagnosed. New approaches include shockwave and infrared-light-source therapies, and new uses have been found for existing therapies. Products have been developed to help treat often painful disorders. Finally, the most revolutionary development in foot care has been cutting-edge surgery, such as the ankle replacement.

The Bad and the Ugly

Not all the changes in foot care in the past few years have been positive. For one thing, I am compelled to speak out against cosmetic plastic surgery of the foot, specifically of the toes. For reasons that I do not fully comprehend, some women and men decide that some or all of their toes are too long and unsightly, even though the digits are functioning well within normal limits and have no deformities. The procedure involves removing a piece of the proximal phalange (the biggest bone in each toe) to shorten the toe. Unfortunately, in many cases this causes a loss of normal motion in the affected toe joint and, in some rare instances, axial rotation (twisting of the toe) after the operation.

Because the foot is acutely sensitive to any changes—even to the toes—the toe-shortening procedure can adversely affect the biomechanics of the foot. I have been a podiatrist for many years, and I will never understand why anyone would have this procedure and risk the complications of surgery to such a crucial part of the body.

In my practice I have yet to meet a patient who feels that his or her life has been adversely affected in any meaningful way because of toes that are too long. Moreover, I have seen many patients—who did have serious deformities preoperatively—for whom foot surgery did not produce the desired effect. A successful outcome is not 100 percent guaranteed for any operation. I want anyone to please think very carefully of the risks involved with any surgery, especially on the feet. You get one pair of feet in your lifetime, and in most cases surgery on them is not reversible. If the operation results in a subsequent foot fault, you will be looking at big trouble down the road. My favorite question to patients who are considering questionable cosmetic foot surgery is, "Should we cut the foot to fit the shoe, or should we cut the shoe to fit the foot?" The answer should be obvious.

What's New in Joints

As people live longer and are therefore more susceptible to extreme wear and tear of weight-bearing joints, hip- and knee-replacement surgery has now become almost commonplace. I expect that as the baby boomers reach retirement age, more and more of them will become candidates for such replacement surgery. Many of them lead very active athletic lives, which increases the risk of joint degeneration—particularly if they run a lot or play sports that place tremendous stresses on the lower extremities.

Since being introduced as a partial solution to the chronic and often acute pain associated with severe osteoarthritis, hip and knee surgeries have come a long way. The latest hip-replacement innovation is "keyhole" surgery, using tiny instruments and different materials. This operation is far less invasive (meaning it requires much smaller incisions), which results in a much shorter hospital stay, less postoperative pain, and a faster recovery period that doesn't require a lengthy stay in a rehab clinic. The patient also loses far less blood than with the traditional procedure, and will definitely not require a blood transfusion. Considering the unpleasant bugs that can lurk in donated blood, despite the best precautions taken by the blood agencies, this new technique is a definite plus. What remains to be seen, however, is the long-term outcome of this surgical procedure. Will the replacement joints last as long as conventional ones? Will there be other, presently unforeseen, complications?

Knee-replacement surgery has also made great strides, as orthopedic surgeons continue to perfect their techniques. I know of an eighty-three-year-old woman who had a successful total knee replace-

ment done two years ago using only epidural freezing. In other words, she was awake during the entire operation, which is an advantage for patients who have medical conditions that may make the use of anesthetics potentially dangerous. In addition, the patient is not as prone to the postoperative nausea commonly associated with administration of anesthetics.

Ankle-replacement surgery was first attempted at least thirty years ago. Unfortunately, the implant materials used then proved unsuccessful, and almost all the total ankle replacements done at that time ultimately failed. The design of the prosthesis implant began to improve in the late 1980s. Thanks to these changes, total ankle-joint replacement has become an available tool for the surgeon to correct severe ankle arthritis. Within the past eight years, ankle-replacement surgery has again been taken seriously by orthopedic reconstructive surgeons. One of the most renowned orthopedic foot and ankle surgeons in the world, Dr. Mark Myerson, is an expert in ankle replacements and has been kind enough to contribute his expertise to this section of the chapter. Dr. Myerson is medical director of the Institute for Foot and Ankle Reconstruction at Mercy Medical Center in Baltimore, Maryland. He has performed well over two hundred ankle replacements.

The ankle joint is extremely complex and, fortunately, very durable, so it is still relatively uncommon to require ankle-replacement surgery for simple osteoarthritic conditions. However, the more baby boomers I see abusing their bodies in an effort to stay in shape, the more I believe that many of them will eventually become candidates for such an operation. Today, the most common reasons for ankle replacements are rheumatoid arthritis, acute trauma to the joint from an accident, or occasionally *osteochondritis dissecans,* in which a piece of bone or cartilage breaks off and causes severe damage to the offended joint.

For people who require ankle-replacement surgery today, the outcomes are generally good—better from a functional standpoint than they would be following an *arthrodesis* procedure. In ankle arthrodesis, the joint is fused or glued together, limiting its up-and-down movement. The main advantage of a total ankle replacement is the return of some freedom of movement in the affected ankle, which is important for walking and exercising. Although full movement of the joint is never wholly regained, even with a total ankle replacement, it is far preferable to the rigidity of a fused ankle. Orthotics may help to improve and control movement of the entire foot after the replacement.

Unfortunately, not all ankle-replacement surgery goes smoothly. Recent scientific reports have indicated that there is a long learning curve for doctors when it comes to this procedure. So if you do need an ankle replacement, make sure that your surgeon has the experience required to operate successfully.

Recovery following a total ankle replacement must be carefully monitored;

rehabilitation and exercise are essential. Dr. Myerson's approach to rehabilitation includes riding an exercise bicycle and therapy in a swimming pool, which begins as soon as the stitches are removed and the incision is healed. These exercises facilitate the range of motion and ultimately improve the final outcome of the joint-replacement procedure.

I wish I could tell you that ankle-replacement surgery comes with a lifetime warranty. However, the procedures and hardware now being used have not been available long enough to be able to determine the long-term outcome. What we can say is that the quality of life of people who have undergone successful ankle replacements has improved dramatically.

I would also like to be able to describe in simple lay terminology how the operation is performed, but the ankle joint is a complex piece of machinery, and the surgery is extremely complicated. However, if you examine Figure 16.1, you will have an idea of what the prosthesis looks like when it has been inserted.

Rheumatoid Arthritis

One of the primary causes of a degenerative ankle joint is rheumatoid arthritis, a disease that can strike people at any age with devastating effect. When it involves the ankle joint, the ideal surgical treatment, if necessary, is total ankle replacement, because damage to the joint is often so severe that there is no other option, and fusion is

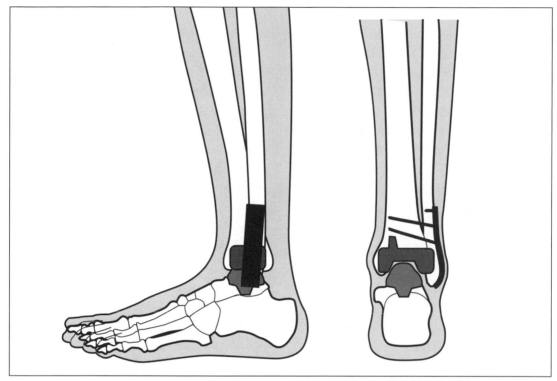

Figure 16.1. Total ankle replacement

not normally the preferred choice. This is because the ankle joint is not the only joint involved at the back of the foot, and it is preferable to maintain as much movement of the foot and ankle as possible. Arthrodesis (fusion) does not provide the desired range of motion.

Rheumatoid arthritis can also have significant effects on other parts of the foot. These range from swelling of the toe joints to severe destruction of the joints. The process of joint inflammation affects the lining (capsule) of the joints first. As the capsule becomes inflamed, the joint fills with fluid and becomes painful. The cartilage lining of the joint may wear out, causing bone to rub on bone. Deformities may

also occur because of loosening of the ligaments and the capsule lining the joint. When this becomes significant, the joints—particularly in the forefoot—may dislocate. In addition, the big toe begins to deviate, causing formation of a bunion.

Obviously, rheumatoid arthritis can create many nasty foot faults, so the ideal situation would be to find a cure for the disease. Unfortunately, there is as yet no magic pill or injection that can rid the body of the condition, although new drugs now on the market can mitigate its effects. However, as is often the case with difficult diseases, the treatments carry their own baggage. The present drugs of choice are extremely expensive and not without side effects, and must be injected rather than administered orally. One of them requires a lengthy intravenous infusion in a clinical setting every eight weeks, after an initial treatment regimen of three doses.

I hope that, by the next time I update this book, a cure for this terrible disease will be available to all sufferers, and will have none of the unpleasant side effects that may accompany the drugs presently used.

Something Old, Something New

Leaving the ankle, we now look a little farther south to the heel, for a new intervention for plantar fasciitis. The treatment is called extracorporeal (outside the body) shockwave therapy, which was born out of a technology called *lithotripsy*. Lithotripsy involves using an extracorporeal shockwave machine to break up very painful kidney stones. These machines send invisible high-energy sound waves through the skin to "blast" the kidney stone, breaking it into hundreds of pieces. The remnants of the stone can then be passed easily with the urine.

It is common in medicine to look at new technologies to see if they can be used for other applications. One of the manufacturers of a lithotripsy machine felt that if it worked for stones, it would probably work for bone spurs as well. The machine manufacturers undertook studies on heel

spurs; to their chagrin, the before and after X rays were the same. However, in a number of cases, although the X ray remained the same, the pain from the plantar fasciitis was reduced and in some cases disappeared completely. The manufacturers quickly prepared their paperwork for FDA approval in the United States to start studies on this phenomenon, not just on heel spurs but also for elbow problems (tennis and golfer's elbow) and some other forms of tendonitis.

This treatment seemed to encourage the tendon and the periosteum to reattach to the underlying bone. Although there are many theories as to why this happens some of the time, no one is exactly sure. A number of leading studies suggest that in medically significant testing (double-blind studies) the placebo effect is actually better than the actual treatment. These studies were so well regarded that most insurance plans in the United States that were considering making this a payable, medically accepted procedure have reduced it to a nonpayable procedure, because it has not been scientifically proven to be medically significant. Personally, I have seen very mixed results with these new machines. In some cases the results were very positive and pain was virtually relieved completely; in the other 40 to 50 percent of patients, there was almost no improvement. Because of the high cost of the treatment, I recommend the tried and tested methods of working to eliminate the major cause of plantar fasciitis—the bad biomechanics—

with orthotics and all the other associated treatments, before you spend the large amount of money for shockwave therapy. I do, however, concede that if all else fails, it is a relatively safe procedure that at worst would have a deleterious effect on your pocketbook.

In the past couple of years there has also been a strong interest in different light therapies, such as cold laser, infrared, and others, that are too plentiful to list here. Sound waves and light therapies have been well recognized for many years in rehabilitation medicine. Depending on whom you talk to and which high-profile personality has been "miraculously cured" by the latest, greatest treatment, you will probably have heard about the treatment flavor of the month.

My comments on these new, improved light and sound-wave therapies are very straightforward. In medicine it is usually not the pen, but the penmanship, that stands the test of time. That is to say, the most important advice is to find and work with a skilled health-care provider who comes highly recommended by other well-regarded practitioners, such as your family doctor, and with whom you have a high level of comfort. This ought to be the single most important part of your treatment plan. When first meeting the practitioner you have chosen to trust with your foot problem, make sure that the diagnosis and treatment program outlined and *all* the alternatives have been thoroughly explained to your satisfaction, and

that you and your practitioner are on the same wavelength as to how you will proceed together.

One of my favorite medical stories is about a surgeon friend who operated on a young lady for bunions. Postoperatively the surgical results were great, but to the patient the operation was an abysmal failure. Why? Because although the doctor removed the bunion and reset the joint exactly as it should have been done, the patient was expecting to go from a size 7E shoe back to a 7AA, which was totally unrealistic. The patient's and the doctor's ideas of success were totally different. So you must always make sure that you and your caregiver are on the same page about expectations, no matter which treatment you decide on together.

Here's a word to the wise about the greatest new treatment for whatever. Medicine is a very old profession, and it stands behind treatments that have stood the test of time for very good reasons. In most cases these treatments (including many "old wives' remedies") carry very little risk, or they would have been discarded, and in the long run they are successful a great deal of the time. With any new product—for example, a motor vehicle—we are always warned not to buy the new model in its first year, but to wait until the manufacturers work out the kinks. Medicine is very similar. The longer a procedure, treatment, or drug has been available, the more time has passed in which to evaluate its efficacy and its side effects.

Chapter 15: The Latest in Noninvasive Care and Foot Surgery

This is not to say that the new noninvasive therapies aren't worth exploring with your medical caregivers. For example, diabetics often have painful feet because of nerve damage, or diabetic neuropathy. Studies are being done to determine whether a spray, using a drug similar to one prescribed for chest pain related to heart disease, might also reduce diabetes-related foot pain. Also, new, improved collagen sponge dressings may promote the healing of diabetes-related foot ulcers. Such dressings are already being used on burn victims to heal areas where skin has been removed for grafting elsewhere on their bodies.

In the final analysis, in medicine you must be wary of claims of 100 percent success. Nothing is 100 percent in medicine—no surgery, no pill, no treatment. Having practiced for almost thirty years now, I can safely argue that our forefathers did so well in medicine in the old horse-and-buggy days because the doctor really got to know the patient and the patient had unbounded trust in the doctor. When I was a young intern, there was a popular TV show called *Marcus Welby, M.D.* In close to an hour (there were fewer commercials in those days), Dr. Welby and his young sidekick would examine, diagnose, and successfully treat a myriad of patients, all of whom he treated as best friends and who adored him in return. That show illustrated the wonderful relationship that can develop between doctor and patient.

Today, for so many different reasons—insurance issues, government regulations, teaching facilities, our helter-skelter lifestyles—those relationships, for the most part, are a thing of the past. Remember that the single most important aspect of treatment is to have trust and faith in your doctor and to work with him or her to maximize the probability of success. Many books have been written by wonderful authors, such as Dr. Bernie Siegel, that expound on how very important this relationship is, especially in our fast-paced modern world. So, before you run out to buy those vibrating shoes to prevent you from losing your balance and falling, or some mass-market inserts that claim to cure all your foot problems, talk to the health-care provider you trust the most. Those products may work, at least for some people, but you could also be throwing away your hard-earned money.

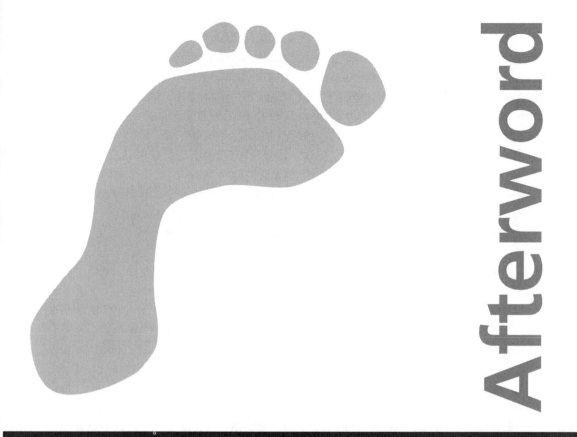

Afterword

Famous Feet
I Have Known

Over my thirty years of practice, I have had the pleasure of treating some of the world's elite athletes and some of the best-known actors and politicians in North America. (By the way, it is often difficult to tell the politicians from the actors.) Although medical ethics prohibit me from discussing patients and their associated problems by name without their consent, I can tell you about some of their problems that I have encountered over the years.

Catching Hell

One of my first professional-athlete patients, who has also become one of my closest friends, was Ernie Whitt, the all-star catcher of the Toronto Blue Jays. When I was asked to join the Blue Jays organization as its foot and ankle consultant in 1980, my first task was to deal with Ernie and his ongoing foot troubles. Consider that, by the young age of twenty-eight, Ernie had caught in over 1,000 professional baseball games, of which more than 350 were at the major league level. Imagine the unbelievable wear and tear on his lower extremities from the awkward position a catcher must maintain for most of the game, crouched behind the plate wearing over twenty pounds of equipment, all resting on the ankle joints. Then imagine jumping up and running after foul balls from that position, not to mention getting hit in the lower extremities by foul tips and, of course, having large players trying to score by running into you at full steam

from third base, attempting to separate your limbs from your torso.

Ernie and I worked very hard together to adjust his footwear and stance with orthotics to alleviate all those awkward pressures and to resolve his ongoing plantar fasciitis. I was a baseball rookie, and Ernie, being a wonderfully friendly but mischievous character, proceeded to play a number of his famous practical jokes on me—such as putting Krazy Glue in my protective rubber gloves, stealing my clothes while I was showering, and altering my expensive suit pants into Bermuda shorts.

Thanks in part to Ernie, my career in baseball mushroomed. I have now examined more than seven hundred baseball players from almost every team, with problems ranging from as simple as a corn to fractures of the lower extremities. I would like to believe that the legacy I am leaving in baseball is one of performance enhancement and injury prevention. Performance enhancement not with drugs, but with methods as simple as my work with a pitcher who had a sore shoulder. He had terrible foot biomechanics, which turned out to be the cause of his shoulder problems. This pitcher is still in the majors after sixteen years and remains one of the best.

At the major-league level, something we might consider to be just one of life's nuisances can become a plague. A very well-known pitcher has yearly ongoing trouble with ingrown toenails on both of his feet. Pitchers often have trouble with ingrown nails because of the stress on the toenails when they "toe off" the mound. (In cases such as this, when I cannot do routine follow-ups, I prefer not to use phenol to kill the nail-growing cells.) On my yearly trips to the spring-training camps in Florida and Arizona, I often have to operate on this wonderful character, who calls me every name under the sun when I freeze his toe and continues to curse and yell the entire time he is completely frozen (feeling absolutely nothing)—just to scare the hell out of the young and often impressionable rookies. Sometimes his bone-chilling screams have actually made the newcomers sick to their stomachs. And, just like a good old fish story that gets repeated (and exaggerated), every year this pitcher tells the rookies that the ingrown nail has gone from just growing into the skin to wrapping around the leg bone and infiltrating all the way up to the hip!

For a rookie, regardless of the sport, training camp can often be traumatic because many of the veterans seem to delight in tormenting them. In 1996, I was at one baseball spring-training camp assessing the foot functions of all the players on the team. The procedure required the players to walk across a computerized mat that records data concerning their gait and determines whether or not they have any foot faults. The veterans decided to have fun with one of the rookies, who was hardly lacking in confidence. They told him that when they walked over the mat they would receive a severe electric shock.

As he stood in line awaiting his turn, the older players began to scream, feigning pain as they walked across the mat. The rookie began to blanch. When it was his turn, he just stood in front of the mat and refused to walk across it. His new teammates pushed him onto the mat, and he screamed before he realized there was no electric shock at all. The veterans howled in enjoyment at their prank. The rookie survived the hazing and has gone on to a successful big-league career.

Of course, major-league sports is a serious business, and with the stresses of performing well come serious injuries. With salaries approaching $25 million a year at the top end, you can extrapolate the cost of losing a player to injury for even one game. In a 162-game season, the top stars are being paid more than $100,000 per game. Pressures on the team medical staff to ensure a safe and quick recovery for each player are very demanding. In my experience, the vast majority of professional players love their respective sports. Just like every Little Leaguer, they can't wait to play, sometimes to the detriment of their well-being. We have only to look back to the 1960s and 1970s in baseball to see how many pro pitching careers ended in their prime, a result of continuing to pitch through injuries at a time when the diagnostic testing and surgical procedures that are the norm today were unavailable. I mentioned earlier that Dizzy Dean injured his great toe and continued pitching through the pain, which eventually caused him to compensate with his pitching arm and led to a permanent shoulder injury that ended his career.

The Sweetest Swing

The most gratifying relationship I have developed in my years of practice is with a very special young man, Shawn Green, who now plays right field for the Los Angeles Dodgers. I first met Shawn in late 1993, a few weeks after the passing of my dad, who had taught me a love of baseball when I was a child growing up in Toronto, a hockey town. Shawn wandered into my life as a fall call-up to the Toronto Blue Jays that year. I had heard all about him, as he was tearing up the minor leagues with his hitting, but had only met him briefly in spring training. On that fateful day our team trainer, Tommy Craig, said he wanted me to examine one of the young rookie call-ups, who had the worst bunions he had ever seen.

In front of me stood a very tall twenty-year-old with two terrible-looking feet. After taking a history and examining his gait, it became obvious that he had tibial varum (was slightly bowlegged) and was developing early wear-and-tear changes in his big-toe joint. Playing half his games on the unforgiving artificial surface of Toronto's SkyDome would only exacerbate the problem.

After I had examined his feet carefully, Shawn stepped into the batting cage for some early extra batting practice. He took a few warm-up swings and then pro-

ceeded to hit nineteen of the coach's twenty-five pitches over the fence, all of them over four hundred feet and one off the glass window of the restaurant far above the center-field wall. In all my years of watching baseball, I had never seen such a mechanically perfect swing, which created a huge challenge for me. How could I help Shawn avoid future foot trouble without changing his beautiful swing? Whatever preventive measures we took would have to preserve that swing. After extensively reviewing videotapes of his swing and analyzing the computerized printouts of his gait, I was able to prescribe an orthotic that simply removed the stresses on his big-toe joint and off-loaded some pressure from the medial side of each knee.

One of my greatest rewards as a podiatrist came in 1998, on the final day of the Blue Jay season. That year, Shawn had already hit twenty-nine home runs, driven in ninety-nine runs, and stolen thirty-five bases. His first two at-bats produced a strikeout and a groundout, but in the seventh inning he smacked a home run into the right-field bleachers. I think I was more excited than Shawn. After the game I walked into the Blue Jays club house, where Shawn was surrounded by the media. In the middle of the press conference, Shawn excused himself, came over, and presented me with the bat and ball that had propelled him to greatness. Those souvenirs are among my most prized possessions.

Yer Out!

In early 2000, I was asked by Mark Letendre, a dear friend who had been head trainer of the San Francisco Giants and had just been appointed medical director for the major-league umpires, to serve as foot and ankle consultant to the umpires. Over the years I had come to know and enjoy the company of many umpires who had been injured while in Toronto. I readily accepted the position and almost immediately set off to umpire spring training. Mark had set up an incredible medical screening program for these men, and my role was to provide expertise in preventing lower-extremity injuries.

Typical baseball fans view umpires as out-of-shape blind men. They may point to the grossly overweight umpire who, on a hot, humid opening day in Cincinnati a few years ago, collapsed behind home plate and died of a heart attack. Today, however, nothing could be further from the truth. The new breed of umpires is, for the most part, just as dedicated to becoming and staying physically fit as most ballplayers. If you don't believe these guys have to be fit, just watch a home-plate umpire stand or crouch awkwardly for three hours, dodging errant hundred-mile-per-hour pitches and foul balls, and sprinting down the third-base line to follow the ball when necessary. (In this category I also include hockey and soccer referees, who often have to race up and down the ice or the field without a break,

and occasionally must officiate games that go long into overtime.)

For many reasons, I do not want to mention by name the umpires I have treated, but they are great patients and dedicated athletes in their own right. Although their jobs place tremendous stress on their lower extremities, almost all of them don their equipment day after day in spite of nagging ankle and foot injuries.

Fore!

Injury prevention and treatment of injury are not all that keep me busy. My expertise in the biomechanics of the lower extremities sometimes leads me to performance-enhancement consultations with a number of highly skilled athletes. Although the majority of the professional athletes I treat are baseball players, I am asked to help athletes from all fields of athletic endeavor.

One of my favorite stories is about the privilege I had three years ago of being summoned by an orthopedic surgeon colleague to examine one of the top golfers in the world, who was suffering from plantar fasciitis. Being a weak weekend golf warrior myself, I couldn't wait to meet and work with this gentleman, hoping, of course, that I would resolve his foot problems and that he would correct my golf swing. Time was of the essence, as it was ten days before one of the four major golf tournaments, and he was rated in the top five. I spent the better part of three hours analyzing his foot plant and reviewing the computerized foot movements during his swing to try to alleviate the abnormal strain on his plantar fascia and possibly to get a somewhat better push-off. We worked through the night making his orthotics so I could work with him on the driving range the next morning. He began his practice swings, and a wide grin spread over his face as he hit his drives more than 325 yards, straight down the middle, every time. In his mind, not only had I markedly reduced his pain, but he was now hitting 10 to 15 yards farther.

I say "in his mind" because one thing I have learned in pro sports is that so much of success or failure is a mind game. I believe, because the pain was reduced and his foot plant was so much stronger, that this golfer was consciously able to get through the ball much better. I had a long discussion with a leading orthopod (orthopedic surgeon) with whom I have worked over the past twenty-five years, Dr. Hamilton Hall. When I queried him about why this may have happened, he said it really didn't matter why it happened as long as the golfer believed it happened. In his years of practice specializing in back pain, he has concluded that much of our success as medical practitioners is based on the positive attitudes of our patients. Dr. Hall once quoted a great sage from many centuries ago who said, "The greatness of a healer can be measured by how well we entertain our patients while mother nature continues to heal." Patients seek our advice for many reasons—one of which is peace of mind. As medical practitioners we often forget that our advice and caring attitude can go miles toward helping our patients heal, and Dr. Hall is a master of this philosophy.

Back to my golfer patient, who went on to lead in the first two days of the tournament. My golfing buddies, who knew I had treated him, harassed me every time we teed off that weekend, because while his shots had become longer and straighter, mine had become shorter and more crooked. Although he did not win, he did place in the top three, which was his highest finish in two years. I still see him on a yearly basis, and he still continues to be one of the best players in the world. I, on the other hand, continue to slice and hook like crazy. His diagnosis of my swing? Try swimming or darts!

Tennis, Anyone?

It is well known that there is a "senior circuit" for professional golfers who have reached an age where they have difficulty outscoring the likes of Tiger Woods or Mike Weir, but who haven't lost their competitive edge (a variation on an old saying that old golfers never die, but they are rarely up to par). Less well known is that from time to time some of the male tennis stars of the 1970s and 1980s also tour. Moreover, they are regulars in the major tournaments, such as Wimbledon and the U.S. Open, that have seniors competitions. In 1999, I was asked to be the foot and ankle consultant for this group of former stars, which included Jimmy Connors, John McEnroe, and Björn Borg.

Although all the players exhibited early wear-and-tear arthritic conditions and some loss of range and motion—remember that a tennis serve places tremendous strain on the forefoot, as do the constant sudden shifts in direction during a rally—I was amazed that they were still able to perform at the highest possible level. All these tennis stars had been extremely careful throughout their careers—and still are when playing—to wear the proper shoes and orthotics. They set an excellent example for all of us baby boomers who want to remain physically active. If you take proper care of your body, you will continue to be able to enjoy your favorite activities.

On Thin Ice

A few years ago I was asked by a trainer for a National Hockey League team to examine a young player who had a severely supinated foot. Because abnormal supination is often associated with a nerve disorder, this player had undergone a complete neurological examination, which indicated no such problem. The team trainer had even experimented with moving the blade of his skate off-center to force him to pronate, but it didn't work.

When I examined the player, I found that he did have a slightly higher arch than normal, but certainly not to the point that it would cause him to supinate so dramatically. But I also discovered that he exhib-ited numbness on the outside of his leg. I asked him if he had suffered some sort of injury to the leg that would cause the numbness. He thought for a long while, then remembered that a few weeks earlier he had been severely slashed from behind during a game. The offending stick had struck him on a part of the leg that wasn't protected by the sophisticated padding worn by hockey players. As a result, he had suffered traumatic nerve damage, specifically, entrapment of the peroneal nerve, which runs down the outside of the leg into the foot. This diagnosis was confirmed by EMG (electromyogram) tests.

A cortisone injection alleviated the nerve entrapment in the player's leg. I also recommended that he wear a modified skate and a special orthotic that would return his foot to a neutral position, so he could pronate and supinate normally. Fortunately, the treatment worked, and the young man is still playing in the National Hockey League.

Dance, Ballerina, Dance

Not all of my stories involve athletes. One of my all-time favorite patients is a ballerina who a few years ago was scheduled to make her National Ballet of Canada lead debut in Tchaikovsky's *The Nutcracker* in Toronto. Today she is one of the top ballerinas in the world, but back then she was a young dancer in distress.

I received an urgent phone call from Dr. Hamilton Hall, who was then the orthopedic consultant to the National Ballet of Canada. This young ballerina had a severely infected, painful big toe caused by a badly ingrown nail, making it virtually impossible for her to dance. Try as she might during rehearsals the day before her debut, whenever she went up on pointe, the excruciating pain made it impossible to continue.

I agreed to see this distraught young lady in my office immediately. She arrived with tears in her eyes and described how the moment she had been preparing for all her life was being destroyed by this infection. She feared that her career was over before it had even begun. After I examined her toe, I realized that the bad infection and offending piece of nail could be easily eliminated, and that she would be able to dance within a couple of days. That was one day too many for her—not good enough. So, after removing the offending piece of nail, I consulted with Dr. Hall and concerned members of the ballet company, and we decided that we could freeze her big toe just before the debut performance so that she could dance. Normally doctors are reluctant to freeze any part of the anatomy to allow strenuous physical activity; the patient could suffer further injury because of not feeling any pain. In the ballerina's case, this was not a major concern, since the infection would heal in time anyway, and the dressing I applied would not be harmed by her dancing.

The ballerina's debut was flawless and received critical acclaim. At the end of the performance she presented my oldest daughter and me with a huge bouquet of roses and thanked me publicly. Later, in her dressing room, she also gave my daughter the ballet slippers she had worn during her performance, which my daughter considers her prize possession to this day. Two weeks later, I received from her one of the nicest letters a doctor could ever receive from a patient. She has since developed into a world-class dancer, and she is also a world-class lady.

The Baritone Sings the Blues

Mark Pedrotti is an opera singer from New Zealand who has been living in Canada for many years. He has sung in opera houses and concert halls around the world. A few years ago he was in Melbourne, Australia, to sing one of the lead roles, Papageno, in Mozart's *The Magic Flute*. There is a scene in the opera in which Papageno is led off the stage blindfolded. At a dress rehearsal, Mark was blindfolded and had begun to walk when he discovered too late that he was much too close to the edge of the stage. When he hit the floor below, one heel took the brunt of the trauma, leaving him with serious soft-tissue damage. Not only did he severely sprain his ankle, he also suffered traumatic tears to the plantar fascia. Fortunately for Mark, the opera house was very close to a sports-medicine facility, and he was expertly treated at once. Thanks to the excellent treatment of the health-care providers there, he was able to sing all his scheduled performances, and the audiences never knew of his discomfort while on stage.

When Mark returned to Toronto a few weeks after the accident, he continued with physiotherapy, although his heel remained quite sore. One of his friends referred him to me for a consultation, as Mark had quite a few performances scheduled and did not want to have to cancel any of them.

After examining Mark's foot, I prescribed an orthotic for his shoe that removed excess pressure from the plantar fascia when he walked. Mark did not have a biomechanical foot fault; in his case, the orthotic was a temporary measure to help his heel recover from the extreme trauma to which it had been subjected in Australia.

Mark wore the orthotic in his shoe for about eighteen months while he slowly healed, during which time he also continued physiotherapy treatments. Once his recovery was complete, he no longer required the insert, and has not had to use orthotics since. Fortunately for him, he suffered no lasting damage to the back of his foot. But he has become much more conscious of where he is standing when he is on the stage.

These are just a few of the better-known patients I have treated in my thirty-plus years as a podiatrist. I wish I could tell you the names of all of them. However, athletes, in particular, are reticent about sharing their medical histories with the general public. Of course, there are times when they are injured in full view of their fans and the media, but normally their foot problems never make the headlines.

Before I conclude, I want to emphasize that, as much as I enjoy treating famous feet, all my patients are special to me. When I am able to successfully treat their problems, I am equally rewarded by their smiles and words of thanks.

Index

A

abduction, 19–20

accessory ossicles, 8

Achilles tendon, 22, 75, 77; in children, 97–98; rupture of, 84, 85. *See also* Achilles tendonitis

Achilles tendonitis, 75, 77; and aerobics, 148; causes of, 82–84; in runners, 137; treatment of, 84–86

acids, as treatment for warts, 71–72

adduction, 20

aerobics, 147–149; shoes for, 192

aging, and foot disorders, 104–108

alcohol consumption, 119–120

alcoholic neuropathy, 120

allergies, 164–165

amputation, 112, 121, 175

amyotrophic lateral sclerosis (ALS), 117

anhidrosis, 169–170

ankle, 8, 21; arthrodesis, 198; and avulsion fracture, 50; joint replacement, 1–2, 97–198; problems for runners, 134–136; and rheumatoid arthritis, 198–200; sprains, 134–135, 149, 151; swollen, 12; taping, 135

anterior compartment syndrome, 139–140

arch, 7, 22–23; in children, 96; fallen, 23; supports for, 25

arteriosclerosis, 11

arthritis, 24–25, 34–35; gonococcal, 116; psoriatic, 116, 167; rheumatoid, 115–116, 198–200

arthrodesis, 198

arthroplasty, 59

aseptic necrosis, 99–100

atherosclerosis, 11, 110

athlete's foot *(tinea pedis)*, 160–164; prevention, 163–164

athletics, 125–126; on artificial turf, 152–153, 156–157; footwear for, 188–193; geriathletes, 104–105; and sports-related injury, 126. *See also* specific sports

Auspitz's sign, 167

autoimmune disorders, 115–116

avulsion fracture, 50

axially rotated toe, 62

B

baby boomers, 2, 104

bacteria, and athlete's foot, 162–163; and foot odor, 168–196

ball (of the foot), 7

baseball, 156–157, 204–207

basketball, 151

biomechanics, abnormal, 16–19, 22–24; and bunions, 31; and calluses, 64–66; congenital abnormalities, 83, 92–95; defined, 15–16; and hammer toes, 53–54; and plantar fasciitis, 77–79; and runners' injuries, 126. *See also* pronation; supination

birth defects, 92–95

blisters, in racket sports, 150; in runners, 127–128

bone scan, 46

bone spurs, 79, 133

bones, avulsion fracture, 50; children's fractures, 99; of the foot, 7–8; navicular, 100; of the rearfoot, 75–76; sesamoids, 46–48; stress fractures, 45–48

Brachman skate, 93, 97, 98

bromidrosis, 169

bunionette, 49–50

bunions, 29–36; baby, 49–50; and biomechanical faults, 31; and calcium levels, 31–32; cause of, 29–32; in children, 98–99; and computer gait analysis, 31; and heredity, 30; and metatarsal-head disorders, 40;

Index

E

edema. *See* swelling
epiphysis (growth plate), 98–99
eversion, 19–20
exercise, for diabetics, 113–114
exostectomy, 49–50, 61
exostosis, 86–87
external tibial torsion, 97

F

fallen arches, 23
flat feet, 23
foot, anatomy of, 6–13; biomechanical fault in, 22–24; bones of, 7–8; and circulation, 11–12; dermatological disorders of, 160–170; fetal development of, 91; functions of, 12–13; joints of, 8–10; muscles of, 10; neuromuscular diseases of, 116–117; during pregnancy, 117–118; size, 6–7; systemic disorders of, 110–123. *See also* specific conditions
football, 152–153
footwear. *See* shoes
forefoot, 7; and abnormal pronation, 21; disorders of, 38–50; injuries in runners, 128–129
forefoot valgus deformity, 47
fractures, avulsion, 50; in children, 99; heel, 76–77; sesamoid bones, 46–48, 129–130; stress, 45–48, 128–129, 148–149
Freiberg's disease, 99–100
friction rubs, 84–85
frostbite, 111, 120–122, 187
fungal infections, 127, 151; antifungal medications, 177; athlete's foot, 160–164; of the toenails, 176–177

G

gait cycle, 16–17; computer analysis of, 1, 22, 26, 44–45
geriatric foot disorders, 104–108
golf, 207–208
Gore, Al, 84
gout, 10, 35, 114–115
Green, Shawn, 206
growth plate, 98–99
gryphotic nails, 151, 177–178
gymnastics, 153

H

Haglund's deformity, 75, 86–87
Hall, Hamilton, 101, 208, 209
hallux limitus, 34–35
hallux rigidus, 34–35
hallux valgus. *See* bunions
hammer toe, causes of, 52–55; in dancers, 150; and the development of corns, 55; in runners, 131; surgery for, 58–59; treatment of, 56–59
heel, Achilles tendonitis, 75, 77; callused, 68–69; and dry skin, 169–170; fracture of, 76–77; plantar fasciitis, 75, 77–82
heel cushions, 81
heel spurs, 79, 133
heloma. *See* corns (heloma)
heredity, and Achilles tendonitis, 83; and bunions, 30–31
hiking, 157–158, 192
hockey, 153–154, 209
home remedies, for calluses, 66–67; for corns, 56–57; dangers of, 56–57, 66–67, 73; for ingrown toenails, 174; for warts, 71–72, 73
hyperhidrosis (excessive perspiration), 169
hypnosis therapy (for warts), 71

Index

161, 176–177; geriatric problems of, 106; gryphotic, 151, 177–178; hygiene, 179–180; ingrown, 151, 173–176, 204–205; problems for dancers, 150–151; problems for runners, 126–127; problems in racket sports, 149–150; psoriatic, 178–179

nerve disorders of the foot, neuroma, 42–45; tarsal tunnel syndrome, 87–89

nerve entrapment, 12, 130–131

nerves, 12

neuroma, 39, 42–45; causes, 42–44; in racket sports, 150; in runners, 130–131; symptoms of, 44; treatment of, 44–45

neuropathy, 111, 112; alcoholic, 120

nucleated callus, 65–66, 67

nutrition, and foot disorders, 110

O

odor, foot, 168–170

onychogryphosis, 177–178

orienteering, 157–158

orthotics, 1, 25–27; for Achilles tendonitis, 85–86; for bunions, 31, 36; for calluses, 67; for children, 98, 100; for neuroma, 44–45; for plantar fasciitis, 81; for skiing, 154; for tarsal tunnel syndrome, 89; for tendonitis, 131; types of, 26

osteoarthritis, 25; and bunions, 34–35; compared to gout, 115; in dancers, 150; of the knee, 143–144; in seniors, 105–106

osteoporosis, 105

osteotomy, 41–42, 49–50

out-toeing, 96–97

overuse syndrome, 148, 158

P

pads, corn, 58

pain, enigmatic, 12; in heel, 77–82; of the knee, 140–143; metatarsal, 39–42. *See also* specific conditions

papilloma virus, 69

Pedrotti, Mark, 210–211

periostitis, 77, 131

perspiration, 168–170

phenol-and-alcohol technique, 174–175

pigeon-toes, 96–97

piriformis syndrome, 145

plantar fasciitis, 75, 77–82; causes of, 77–79; in dancers, 151; and racket sports, 149; in runners, 133–134; shockwave therapy, 200–201; symptoms of, 79–80; treatment of, 80–82, 133–134

plantar flexion, 20, 39; symptoms of, 39–41

plantar set procedure, 58–59

plantar warts. *See* warts

podagra. *See* gout

podopediatrics, 91

polio (poliomyelitis), 116–117

pregnancy, 117–118

pronation, 8–9; abnormal, 1, 20–22; and chondromalacia patella, 141; and the gait cycle, 17–20; and knee problems, 142–143; and metatarsal-head disorders, 40; and plantar fasciitis, 80–81; in runners, 139, 141–142, 144

psoralen drugs, 168

psoriasis, 166–168, 178–179

psoriatic arthritis, 167

psuedo-gout, 114

pumice stones, 58

pump bump (Haglund's deformity), 86–87

pustular psoriasis, 167

PUVA therapy, 168

R

racket sports, 133, 149–150, 208–209; shoes for, 191–192

ram's horn nail, 178

Index

93; for corns, 58–59, 61–62; cosmetic, 196;
endoscopic, 82; exostectomy, 61; for fractured sesamoids, 129; for fungal infection
of the toenail, 177; for Haglund's deformity, 87; for hammer toes, 58–59; for
ingrown toenails, 174–175; joint replacement, 196–198; keyhole, 197; for knee
pain, 101; laser, 73; for metatarsal-head
pain, 41; minimal incision (MIS), 50, 59,
175; for neuroma, 45; for plantar fasciitis,
81–82; for varicose veins, 119; for warts,
72–73

sweat glands, 168–170
swelling, of the ankle, 12; and neuroma, 43;
and plantar flexion, 39–40; and tarsal tunnel syndrome, 88; when traveling, 119
swing phase (gait), 17
sympathectomy, 169
synovitis, 39, 136
systemic arthritic diseases, 25

T

talipes valgus (club foot), 92–93
talipes varus (club foot), 92–93
tarsal tunnel syndrome, 75, 87–89, 136
tarsus, 75. *See also* ankle; rearfoot
tea tree oil, 162
tendonitis, 10, 131–133
tendons, 10
tennis, 133, 208–209
therapy, for Achilles tendonitis, 84–85; laser,
41, 135, 175–176, 201; ultraviolet-ray,
167–168
tobacco, 119–120
toenails. *See* nails
toes, baby, 49–50, 62; big-toe joint, 10;
bunions, 29–36; claw toes, 53; gout, 10, 35,

114–115; hammer toe, 52–55; injuries to
soccer players, 156; mallet toes, 53; over-
lapped, 94; supernumerary, 94; surgery to
align, 33–34; turf toe, 152–153, 156; walking on, 97–98
tracks, indoor, 135–136
trainer, athletic, 158
tumor (neuroma), 42–45
turf toe, 152–153, 156

U

ulcers, skin, 111, 112
ultrasound, 1, 41, 46, 80, 131, 201
ultraviolet-ray therapy, 167–168
uric acid, 114, 115

V

varicose veins, 12, 118–119
vasoconstriction, 119–120
vasodilation, 119
veins of the leg, 11–12; varicose veins, 12,
118–119
venereal disease, 116
verruca vulgaris, 69
volleyball, 151

W

walking, 105
walking cycle, 16–17
warts, compared to calluses, 64; freezing, 72;
home remedies for, 71–72, 73; plantar,
69–70; removal of, 70–71; surgery for,
72–73; types of, 69
webbed feet, 94
Whitt, Ernie, 204

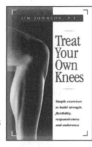
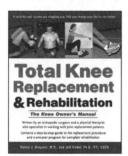
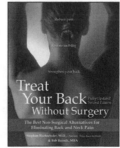

THE CHIROPRACTOR'S SELF-HELP BACK AND BODY BOOK:
How You Can Relieve Common Aches and Pains at Home and on the Job

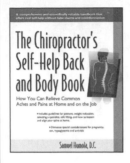

by Samuel Homola, D.C.

Written by a chiropractor with over 40 years experience, this book is for people with chronic head, neck, arm, wrist, back, hip, leg, and shoulder pain as well as sufferers from osteoporosis, a weak back, sciatica, arthritis, and hypoglycemia. It includes information on how to handle arthritis, how to protect a weak back during sex and pregnancy, and how to tell sense from nonsense in the chiropractic care of your back pain. The book is illustrated with 42 line drawings prepared by a professional artist.

320 pages ... 42 illus. ... Paperback $17.95

SHAPEWALKING: Six Easy Steps to Your Best Body ... *Second Edition*
by Marilyn Bach, Ph.D., and Lorie Schleck, M.A., P.T.

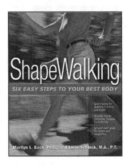

Millions of Americans want an easy, low-cost fitness program. *ShapeWalking* is the answer. It includes aerobic exercise, strength training, and flexibility stretching and is ideal for exercisers of all levels who want to control weight; develop muscle definition; prevent or reverse loss of bone density; and spot-shape the stomach, buttocks, arms, and thighs. The second edition includes over 70 photographs as well as updated exercises and resources.

144 pages ... 73 photos ... Paperback $14.95

GET FIT WHILE YOU SIT: Easy Workouts from Your Chair
by Charlene Torkelson

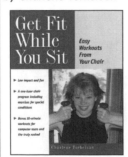

Here is a total-body workout that can be done right from your chair, anywhere. It is perfect for office workers, travelers, and those with age-related movement limitations or special conditions. This book offers three programs. The One-Hour Chair Program is a full-body, low-impact workout that includes light aerobics and exercises to be done with or without weights. The 5-Day Short Program features five compact workouts for those short on time. Finally, the Ten-Minute Miracles is a group of easy-to-do exercises perfect for anyone on the go.

160 pages ... 212 photos ... Paperback $14.95

Prices subject to change without notice

THE CORTISOL CONNECTION: Why Stress Makes You Fat and Ruins Your Health — and What You Can Do About It ... *by Shawn Talbott, Ph.D.*

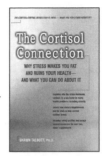

Cortisol is the primary stress hormone, activated by the fight-or-flight stress response. Research has shown a close connection between chronic stress, high cortisol levels, and serious health problems such as obesity, diabetes, hypertension, and depression.

The Cortisol Connection explains the health risks of high cortisol and the contains the author's SENSE program (Stress management; Exercise; Nutrition; Supplementation; Evaluation) for controlling cortisol levels and managing weight gain.

288 pages ... 7 illus. ... 21 tables ... Paperback $15.95

THE CORTISOL CONNECTION DIET: The Breakthrough Program to Control Stress and Lose Weight
by Shawn Talbott, Ph.D., FACSM

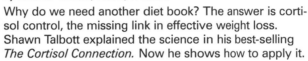

Why do we need another diet book? The answer is cortisol control, the missing link in effective weight loss. Shawn Talbott explained the science in his best-selling *The Cortisol Connection.* Now he shows how to apply it.

This pocket-sized guide explains how to eat for quality at every meal to achieve *healthy* weight loss, how to use dietary supplements and exercise to control cortisol and blood sugar, and how to change your metabolic response to food and lose those last 10 pounds. Sample plans for meals, snacks, and supplements are included.

144 pages ... 12 illus. ... 21 tables ... Paperback $8.95

SPORTS NUTRITION FOR WOMEN ... *Second Edition*
Anita Bean, B.Sc., and Peggy Wellington, B.Sc., M.Phil., Editors

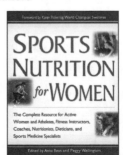

Women who exercise regularly may encounter problems that could be prevented by better nutrition. This thoroughly researched book examines the specific nutritional requirements of active women and offers condensed information and advice. Each chapter is written by a specialist and covers topics such as body fat and weight management, iron and sports anemia, bone health, and nutrition for team sports and during pregnancy.

192 pages ... 15 illus. ... 32 tables ... Paperback $15.95

To order or for our FREE catalog call (800) 266-5592

ORDER FORM

NAME

ADDRESS

CITY/STATE   ZIP/POSTCODE

PHONE   COUNTRY (outside of U.S.)

TITLE	QTY	PRICE	TOTAL
The Good Foot Book		@ $16.95	
Treat Your Own Knees		@ $10.95	

Prices subject to change without notice

Please list other titles below:

		@ $	
		@ $	
		@ $	
		@ $	
		@ $	

Check here to receive our book catalog ☐   *FREE*

Shipping Costs:
By Priority Mail, first book $4.50, each additional book $1.00
By UPS and to Canada, first book $6.00, each additional book $2.00
For rush orders and other countries call us at (510) 865-5282

TOTAL   _____
Less discount @ _____ %   (_____)
TOTAL COST OF BOOKS   _____
Calif. residents add 7½ sales tax   _____
add Shipping & handling   _____
TOTAL ENCLOSED   _____
Please pay in U.S. funds only

☐ Check   ☐ Money Order   ☐ Visa   ☐ MasterCard   ☐ Discover

Card # _____ Exp. date _____

Signature _____

Complete and mail to:
Hunter House Inc., Publishers
PO Box 2914, Alameda CA 94501-0914
Phone (510) 865-5282 Fax (510) 865-4295
You can also order by calling **(800) 266-5592**
of from **www.hunterhouse.com**

GFB 11/2004